The Menopause Cookbook

The Menopause Cookbook

How to Eat Now and for the Rest of Your Life

Hope Ricciotti, M.D., and
Vincent Connelly

W. W. Norton & Company

New York | London

For information about permission to reproduce selections from this book,
write to Permissions, W. W. Norton & Company, Inc.,
500 Fifth Avenue, New York, NY 10110

The text of this book is composed in Adobe Garamond
with the display set in Mona Lisa Recut and Solid
Composition by Gina Webster
Manufacturing by Courier Companies
Book design by Chris Welch

Library of Congress Cataloging-in-Publication Data

Ricciotti, Hope.
The menopause cookbook : how to eat now and for the rest of your life /
Hope Ricciotti and Vincent Connelly.
p.   cm.
Includes index.
ISBN 0-393-31983-0 (pbk.)
1. Menopause—Nutritional aspects. 2. Cookery.
I. Connelly, Vincent. II. Title.
RG186.R48   2000
612.6'65—dc21   99–34029
CIP

W. W. Norton & Company, Inc., 500 Fifth Avenue, New York, N.Y. 10110
www.wwnorton.com

W. W. Norton & Company Ltd., 10 Coptic Street, London WC1A 1PU
1 2 3 4 5 6 7 8 9 0

For Joe and Leo

Contents

Part 2 Recipes

The
Menopause
Cookbook

Introduction

Menopause is an important phase in the life cycle of all women, one that only recently has captured our attention. More than one-third of a woman's life is spent during and after menopause. Maintaining a healthy and active lifestyle appropriate to the new requirements of your body will maximize your enjoyment of this phase of your life. While some women find the passage through menopause difficult, others find it a welcome change. Many of my patients come to me with great relief that they no longer have to deal with monthly menstruation or worries about birth control. For some, though, hot flashes, sleep disturbances, irritability, and vaginal dryness make this time a trying one. In addition, many women become increasingly worried about diseases that are more common during menopause: heart disease, osteoporosis, and breast cancer.

You can reduce your risk of disease and maximize your energy and health through eating a healthy diet, getting enough exercise, and replacing the estrogen your body now lacks. The replacement of estrogen can be accomplished through diet by consuming plant sources of estrogens (phytoestrogens) or by using a hormone replacement therapy.

Health Maintenance While it is important throughout your life to maintain good health, it is particularly important in menopause. After menopause the bones begin to thin, heart disease becomes more common, and many cancers have their peak incidence. Many of these problems can be prevented by straightforward adjustments in diet and lifestyle. In fact, improving one's diet, maintaining exercise programs, not smoking, minimizing alcohol intake, and reducing stress do more to keep you healthy than all the medicines and doctors in the world can do.

Medicalization of Menopause Many women have reacted against the so-called medicalization of menopause. Hormone replacement therapy has been promoted as a cure to many of the ills of menopause. Some women feel very comfortable taking hormone replacement therapy and have minimal side effects. However, many women have problems with it philosophically or physically. Some feel that it does not make intuitive sense to them that a natural part of the life cycle should require taking pills. Others have terrible side effects or medical problems that prevent them from being able to take such therapies. The diverse needs of women in menopause should be respected and tailored to each individual. There is no one right way for everyone.

A Moderate's Approach As a physician dealing with a heterogeneous population of women, with varying risk factors for heart disease, breast cancer, and osteoporosis, I am faced daily with helping women make good decisions about what is right for them in menopause. My one goal is to maximize their health and wellness during menopause. For some women hormone replacement therapy is the best answer. For others taking hormone replacement therapy is detrimental to their health or unacceptable to their philosophies. In order to respect the needs of all these women, I arm myself with as many alternatives as possible. For some women I prescribe traditional hormone replacement therapy. For others we discuss dietary changes to enhance their intake of estrogens through food sources. For all women I encourage a low-fat, high-fiber, antioxidant-rich diet, and regular exercise.

Diet and Menopause Phytoestrogens, plant sources of estrogen, have been receiving a great deal of publicity as an alternative to taking synthetic hormones during menopause. They have been shown to confer similar health benefits on the body while also preventing some of the uncomfortable symptoms of menopause. Unlike hormone replacement therapy, they appear to decrease the risk of breast and other cancers and do not have side effects. Best of all, they can be incorporated into a diet that is healthy, low fat, and delicious. All women, whether they are taking hormone replacement therapy or not, can benefit from a diet rich in phytoestrogens. In addition, such a diet can be tailored to be heart-healthy, rich in antioxidants to fight cancer, quick to prepare, and appealing to the whole family.

A Cookbook for Menopause Eating well in menopause can be simple and delicious. Phytoestrogens are not typically part of the American diet, being found in large amounts in flaxseed and soy foods: tofu, tempeh, miso, and soy milk. Since soy foods and their preparation are unfamiliar to the average American, this book is designed to incorporate them into cooking in easy and delicious ways. Tofu does not need to be only for vegetarians. It can be incorporated into a varied diet in appealing ways. In addition, silken tofu can be hidden as a substitute for cream in many recipes, turning high-fat recipes into heart-healthy and phytoestrogen-rich ones. My husband, the chef Vincent Connelly, and I had a great deal of fun creating these unique, simple, and good-tasting recipes targeted toward the mainstream woman, who is concerned about her health, interested in eating well, and open to new possibilities in cooking.

This book is about health and wellness through lifestyle changes in menopause and perimenopause. Dietary adaptations during menopause can prevent many of the major causes of ill health in our society today. Eating well not only is good for your health but also can be enjoyable, easy, and fun for the whole family.

Part 1

❖

Menopause, Health, and Nutrition

Chapter 1

What Is Menopause?

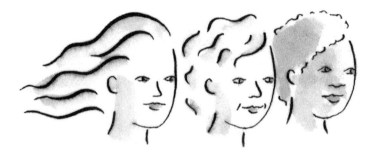

Menopause and the Female Life Cycle

Menopause is a major landmark in the life cycle of a woman, marking the time when childbearing is over and a new phase of life begins. Since the average age of menopause is approximately 52 years and the average life expectancy for a woman is about 78 years, more than one-third of your life will be spent after menopause. It is therefore important to take measures to maximize your health and wellness to accommodate your body's new needs. Much can be accomplished through diet, exercise, and lifestyle changes.

The transition through menopause can last a few months to

a few years. During this time your body senses a decrease in the amount of estrogen produced from the ovary. This decrease causes the symptoms of menopause that many women notice: irregular periods, hot flashes, mood disturbances, and vaginal dryness. Eventually, the ovary stops producing estrogen entirely, a time known as postmenopause. Most women are no longer as symptomatic during their postmenopausal years.

Age at Menopause The age in which you enter menopause is predetermined genetically. Your age at menopause is not related to the number of times you previously ovulated or had your period. It is not affected by the number or timing of any previous pregnancies or breastfeeding. It is not affected by the use of oral contraceptives or lack of regular ovulation. However, certain lifestyle or health issues may slightly affect menopause. In studies cigarette smokers have been shown to experience an earlier spontaneous menopause than nonsmokers.

Menopause and Hormones

Menopause Defined Menopause is defined as the permanent cessation of your period (menstruation) caused by loss of egg development in the ovary. The basic feature of menopause is that the ovary becomes depleted of eggs, and the cells surrounding the eggs no longer respond to hormonal stimulation by producing estrogen. Thus a new hormonal state arises in your body postmenopausally, one characterized by low estrogen levels, the loss of which affects many organ systems and structures in your body.

Hormone Regulation in Menopause Before menopause the hormones FSH (follicle stimulating hormone) and LH (luteinizing hormone) are produced in the pituitary gland in the brain and flow through the blood to stimulate egg development in the ovary. After the release of the egg from the ovary (ovulation), the ovary produces a great deal of estrogen, which circulates to the rest of the body through the blood and nourishes many body tissues.

Once menopause occurs and ovulation ends, the whole process stops, and estrogen is no longer produced in the ovary. The pituitary gland senses the low estrogen level in the blood and sends out more FSH and LH to try to stimulate the ovary to produce an egg. But the ovary is depleted of eggs and cannot respond by producing an egg or any more estrogen. Your periods get lighter and further apart and eventually stop completely. You sense the loss of estrogen in your body with such symptoms as hot flashes, vaginal dryness, urinary frequency, fatigue, and irritability. Blood levels of FSH and LH are very high at this time, which is how menopause can be diagnosed by a blood test. Elevated blood FSH levels, above 20 pg/ml, confirm menopause has begun. (LH is not as reliable a blood test for menopause as FSH because it can become elevated just before ovulation.) Most women do not require a blood test to diagnose menopause. The loss of your monthly period and associated symptoms such as hot flashes and vaginal dryness can confirm this new stage of the life cycle.

This whole process can begin up to five years before actual menopause. During this time FSH levels increase, and estrogen levels begin to decrease even though the menstrual cycles remain ovulatory—that is, release an egg. The decrease in estrogen before actual menopause accounts for the fact that some women will have hot flashes during the five years before their periods stop completely.

Hormones Produced after Menopause The ovary is not totally inactive postmenopausally. The cells surrounding the eggs in the ovary continue to produce male hormones known as androgens—testosterone and androstenedione. Androgens are converted to estrogens in the body fat. Therefore, women who have larger fat stores will convert more of these male hormones into estrogen and ultimately have higher blood levels of estrogen than thin women. For that reason overweight women are less likely to develop symptoms of estrogen deficiency (such as hot flashes and vaginal dryness) and osteoporosis. Slim women are more likely to experience hot flashes, since they do not have much body fat and are therefore not converting much of their androgens into estrogen. Thin women are also at an increased risk for osteoporosis.

Physical, Emotional, and Psychological Effects of Menopause

Effects of Low Estrogen Levels on the Body During the years before menopause, the main source of estrogen in your body is the eggs in the ovary. Once menopause begins, the estrogen levels in your blood decline rapidly, and your body will sense the decrease. Symptoms will occur in many body tissues as a consequence of these low levels of estrogen. Some women will experience multiple severe symptoms, while others have minimal reactions.

Irregular bleeding. Disturbances in menstrual patterns, with either decreased or increased flow, can occur. Ovulation, the release of the egg from the ovary, is what triggers your period, approximately two weeks later. When you do not ovulate, the signals for the release and breakdown of the lining of the uterus do not occur. The lining gradually builds up and eventually outgrows its blood supply, causing it to slough off irregularly. This causes irregular spotting (light bleeding). You may also ovulate less frequently, perhaps only every two to four months. These infrequent periods can be quite heavy, since the uterine lining may have built up during this time. Overweight women tend to have the most trouble with heavy bleeding, because other hormones (androgens) are converted to a weak form of estrogen (estrone) in fatty tissues, and the estrogen can cause the uterine lining to build up over time.

Vaginal dryness. Approximately 25 percent of menopausal women notice vaginal dryness, sometimes as quickly as a few months after menopause begins. You may also notice vaginal discharge, itching, burning, light bleeding from the vagina, and pain with intercourse. All of these symptoms can be caused by the effect of low estrogen levels on the vaginal tissues.

Hormone replacement therapy will relieve vaginal dryness effectively. Alternative treatments to hormonal therapy include consuming more soy products although the exact amount it takes to prevent dryness has not yet been determined. In addition, effective vaginal lubricating products are available, such as water-based jellies, creams, or oils, that help many women. Finally, less vaginal atrophy seems to occur in women who are more sexually active, that is, who have intercourse three or more times per month.[1]

Hot flashes. Hot flashes are considered the defining symptom of menopause. A hot flash is a sudden, explosive phenomenon lasting three to four minutes characterized by a feeling of heat in the skin, especially the face. Physiologically, both blood flow to the extremities and skin temperature increase. Hot flashes frequently occur at night, awakening you from sleep and then producing insomnia. This sleep deprivation leads to irritability and moodiness. Hot flashes do not persist in most women for more than two to three years.

Hot flashes are caused by decreased estrogen levels in the blood. The change in estrogen levels leads to alterations in the central nervous system, causing the hot flashes to occur. The more sudden the onset of low estrogen levels (such as after surgical removal of the ovaries) or the younger you are when you experience menopause, the more severe the hot flashes are. About 75 percent of women in the United States going through menopause develop hot flashes. Women who are overweight tend to have a smaller drop in estrogen levels and are therefore less likely to have severe hot flashes.

Soy in the diet has been shown definitively to decrease the incidence of hot flashes. Sixty grams (approximately two

[1]S. Leiblum, G. Bachmann, E. Kemmann, et al. Vaginal atrophy in the postmenopausal woman. *Journal of the American Medical Association* 249: 2195, 1983.

ounces) of soy protein daily results in a 45 percent reduction in hot flashes.[2] Hormone replacement therapy will reduce the occurrence of hot flashes. Regular exercise may reduce hot flashes. They are triggered by such stimuli as caffeine, alcohol, spicy foods, hot weather, emotional distress, or even a warm room. Avoiding these situations can reduce hot flashes.

Mood disturbances. Many women find that their moods become unpredictable during menopause. Symptoms such as anxiety, depression, irritability, and fatigue can increase during this time. Controversy exists as to whether estrogen deficiency directly causes these symptoms or whether hot flashes causing insomnia result in sleep deprivation and indirectly cause the mood disturbances. Most experts believe that mood disturbances in menopause result from sleep deprivation caused by hot flashes. Currently no evidence exists that menopause directly causes depression or that menopause is associated with increased rates of depression. However, women with a previous history of depression, postpartum depression, or severe premenstrual syndrome may be at increased risk for depression at menopause.

Insomnia is usually a direct result of hot flashes, although it may arise because of other effects of estrogen deprivation. Treatments for hot flashes therefore will usually result in a better quality of sleep. Another natural remedy for insomnia is warm milk taken before bedtime because it is a source of the amino acid tryptophan. Tryptophan is metabolized into serotonin in the brain. Enhanced serotonin levels in the brain are associated with relief of pain and depression and better quality of sleep. Exercise also has a beneficial effect on the quality of sleep. In physically fit individuals, the amount of deep sleep is higher. In addition, after three months of regular exercise, a mood-enhancing effect of exercise takes place, correlating with a higher level of fitness. Most experts recommend that if insomnia and moodiness do not respond to these measures, then treatment for depression should be considered.

[2] P. Albertazzi, F. Pansini, B. Bonacorsi, et al. The effect of dietary soy supplementation on hot flushes. *Obstetrics and Gynecology* 91: 6, 10, 1998.

Healthy Body, Healthy Mind A word about mental health: In addition to keeping the body healthy, it is also important to keep your mind healthy. Depression and anxiety can be common problems in women at any time in the life cycle. It is important to recognize and treat these problems, just as it is important to treat physical problems. I often remind women who seek my attention for medical issues, but really are suffering from depression or anxiety, that the mind needs as much, if not more, attention as the body in order to maintain health. After all, wouldn't you take insulin if you had diabetes? So why wouldn't you accept treatment for depression or anxiety?

As preventive therapy for good mental health, keep stress to a minimum, simplify your life, learn mind/body relaxation techniques, and accept mental-health support when needed. These ways of keeping the mind healthy are all equally as important as taking care of your body for wellness during and after menopause.

Menopause and Alzheimer's Disease No evidence suggests that the loss of estrogen at menopause increases the risk of Alzheimer's disease. However, some preliminary data show hormone replacement therapy may help prevent that devastating disease. It is too early to determine if phytoestrogens will confer similar benefits.

Menopause and Osteoporosis Osteoporosis is a disease in which the skeleton thins, causing the bones to become fragile, which leads to an increased risk of bone fractures. Bone health is influenced by three major interacting factors: diet, exercise, and estrogen. Because estrogen protects your bones from thinning, osteoporosis becomes much more common after a woman goes through menopause.

Preventing osteoporosis begins with good dietary levels of calcium and plenty of weight-bearing exercise. Several medical interventions can prevent osteoporosis or treat it in its early stages: calcium supplementation, hormone replacement therapy, and drugs that act directly on the bones to prevent bone loss. Soy in the diet shows some promise in preventing osteo-porosis, but it has not yet been definitively proven (see Chapter 5, Preventing Osteoporosis).

Menopause and Heart Disease Arteriosclerosis (hardening of the coronary arteries of the heart) is the most common cause of death in women. It becomes much more common after menopause, since the estrogen produced by the body before this time has a protective effect on the heart. After menopause estrogen deficiency leads to higher LDL cholesterol (bad cholesterol) and lower HDL cholesterol (good cholesterol). The overall effect is a more unfavorable lipid profile thought to contribute to the development of arteriosclerosis. In addition to the lipid changes, estrogens have a direct effect on blood vessel walls. Estrogen promotes relaxation of blood vessel walls, allowing them to remain open and not clogged with atherosclerosis.

The development of heart disease in women can be prevented in many individuals. Your diet should be low in fat and rich in phytoestrogens. You and your health-care provider should consider whether some form of hormone replacement therapy is right for you. In addition, you should incorporate regular exercise, weight control, blood pressure control, and smoking cessation into your approach to preventing heart disease.

Menopause, a Positive Experience Although the adverse symptoms of menopause are cited frequently, most women do not find it to be a negative experience. The Massachusetts Women's Health Study, one of the largest and most comprehensive studies of middle-aged women, provides a powerful argument that menopause is not and should not be viewed as a negative experience by the vast majority of women.[3] The

[3]S. M. McKinlay and J. B. McKinlay. The impact of menopause and social factors on health. In C. B. Hammond, F. P. Haseltine, and I. Schiff, eds., *Menopause: Evaluation, Treatment and Health Concerns* (New York: Alan R. Liss, 1989), pp. 137–61.

women studied perceived menopause as having almost no impact on subsequent physical and mental health, and they expressed either positive or neutral feelings about menopause.

Menopause is not always a dramatic, uncomfortable time. While some women are troubled by symptoms related to the loss of estrogen, many women I care for notice only the gradual cessation of their periods. Often, it can be a relief to no longer worry about monthly menstruation or pregnancy. Women who have experienced painful periods, pain from fibroids, or severe premenstrual syndrome often can find that menopause cures them of the symptoms caused by these problems. While about three-quarters of women will suffer from hot flashes, that leaves one-quarter who will not have these symptoms at all. Some women find hot flashes to be very mild and barely noticeable. For these individuals the passage through menopause is not dramatic, with only the loss of their monthly menses to mark it.

Women with more troublesome symptoms have many alternatives in therapy to choose from. Selecting what is right for you depends on your symptoms and your personal risk factors for heart disease and different types of cancer. Educating yourself about the options in menopause will allow you to have a productive relationship with your health-care provider so that you may maximize your health and wellness during and after menopause.

Chapter 2

Phytoestrogens

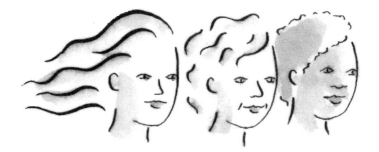

Dietary Answers to Estrogen Loss

Menopause is a time when your body stops producing its own estrogen. Many of the discomforts of menopause—hot flashes, mood disturbances, sleep difficulties, fatigue, vaginal dryness—are related to this lack of estrogen. These are short-term discomforts associated with the onset of menopause. In some women these symptoms last a few months, while in others they can last a few years. Eventually, when you become post-menopausal, they do go away. However, sometimes the vaginal dryness persists. In addition to these short-term discomforts, women also have long-term health risks associated with the lack of estrogen after menopause: an increased risk of heart disease, osteoporosis, and possibly Alzheimer's disease.

It is therefore important that you replace the estrogen your body now lacks. While some women do so through hormone replacement therapy, other women may prefer to replace estrogen by eating plant compounds known as phytoestrogens. Phytoestrogens are substances that occur naturally in plants, especially in soybeans and flaxseed. This form of dietary estrogen is a newly recognized alternative to hormone-replacement therapy. It can be incorporated as part of a heart-healthy, low-fat diet that is good for all individuals, menopausal or not, female or male. It appears that phytoestrogens not only help menopausal symptoms but also may protect from many cancers, including breast cancer, making phytoestrogens even more important during and after menopause.

What Are Phytoestrogens? Phytoestrogens are compounds that are found in plants and have activity similar to estrogen in the body. The chemical makeup of phytoestrogens resembles your own body's estrogen. Because of that resemblance phytoestrogens can mimic the action of your natural estrogen on your body's tissues and organs. Most phytoestrogens are relatively weak estrogens, but they can have significant effects on the body when they are eaten regularly. They have been proven to decrease hot flashes[1] and may have an effect on other symptoms of menopause, including mood disturbances, sleep difficulties, fatigue, and vaginal dryness. Whether phytoestrogens will also protect you from the long-term detrimental health effects of the loss of estrogen at menopause—osteoporosis and heart disease—is currently being investigated and appears promising.

The Chemistry of Phytoestrogens in the Body In humans, after consumption of phytoestrogens from plants, complex chemical reactions occur in the gastrointestinal tract, resulting in the formation of compounds with a close similarity in structure to estrogen. After consumption of soy foods or flaxseed, phyto-

[1]P. Alvertazzi, F. Pansini, and G. Bonaccorsi. The effect of dietary soy supplementation on hot flushes. *Obstetrics and Gynecology* 91: 6–11, 1998.

estrogen metabolites can be measured in the urine, plasma, feces, semen, bile, saliva, and breast milk, showing that the compounds are absorbed from the plants and used in the body.

Concentrations of phytoestrogens in the body can vary widely between individuals even when a controlled quantity of phytoestrogen is administered. Studies have found that many factors, including dietary fiber and vegetable and fruit intake, influence the metabolism of phytoestrogens. Macrobiotics and other vegetarians, such as Seventh Day Adventists, have the highest excretion values of phytoestrogen metabolites. Thus, combining phytoestrogen-rich foods with lots of fruits and vegetables will maximize your benefits.

Food Sources of Phytoestrogens Foods that have high levels of phytoestrogens are soy foods and flaxseed. Phytoestrogens can be divided into two major classes: isoflavones and lignans. Soy foods are rich in isoflavones, while flaxseed is rich in lignans. In addition, small amounts of phytoestrogens in the form of lignans are found in lentils, dried seaweed, wheat, garlic, asparagus, and squash, but the amounts are tiny compared with those in soy foods and flaxseed. Soy products available in the United States include soy milk, tofu, texturized vegetable protein (TVP), and tempeh.

PHYTOESTROGEN CONTENT FROM LIGNANS[2]

Food	Total (mg/4 oz serving)
Flaxseed meal	77.0
Flaxseed flour	60.0
Lentils	1.8
Dried seaweed	2.5
Soybeans	0.9
Wheat	1.0
Garlic	0.5
Asparagus	0.5
Squash	0.5

[2] J. Blake. Phytoestrogens: The food of menopause? *Journal of the Society of Obstetricians and Gynecologists of Canada*, May 1998.

PHYTOESTROGEN CONTENT FROM ISOFLAVONES[3]

Food	Total (mg/4 oz serving)
Roasted soybeans	185
Texturized vegetable protein	157
Soyflour	154
Tempeh	128
Tofu	71

The Soy Alternative

Japanese Women and Menopause The evidence pointing toward phytoestrogens as a possible dietary alternative for treatment of menopausal symptoms came initially from Asia. Asian populations, such as those in Japan, Taiwan, and Korea, are estimated to consume 20 to 150 milligrams a day (with an average of 40 a day) of phytoestrogens from isoflavones in tofu and miso.[4] To give you an idea of how much tofu that would be, 2.25 ounces of tofu contain 40 mg of isoflavones. Although that does not seem like much tofu, it is still a much higher amount than a typical American eats in a day, since Americans often do not consume any soy products. Population studies of Japanese women going through menopause indicate that less than 25 percent suffer from hot flashes,[5] compared with 85 percent of North American women.[6]

[3]J. Blake. Phytoestrogens: The food of menopause? *Journal of the Society of Obstetricians and Gynecologists of Canada*, May 1998.

[4]A. C. Eldridge and F. Kwolek. Soybean isoflavones: Effect of environment and variety on composition. *Journal of Agricultural and Food Chemistry* 31: 394–96, 1983.

[5]M. Lock. *Encounters with Aging: Mythologies of Menopause in Japan and North America* (Berkeley and Los Angeles: University of California Press, 1993).

[6]M. Notelovitz. Estrogen replacement therapy indications, contraindications, and agent selection. *American Journal of Obstetrics and Gynecology* 161: 8–17, 1989.

Perhaps even more important, Japanese women eating a traditional diet rich in soy products have a low incidence of estrogen-dependent cancers, such as breast cancer,[7] compared with Western women. That incidence increases once Asian women westernize their diet.[8] Breast, colon, prostate, endometrial, and ovarian cancers and coronary heart disease all have lower incidence rates in Asia and eastern Europe than in Western countries.[9] Japan consistently has been reported to have the lowest risk of hormone-dependent cancers.[10]

How much soy is the right amount? No one knows the answer to this question. The average Asian woman's diet contains about 3 to 4 ounces of soy foods, such as tofu, a day, yielding about 25 to 40 milligrams of isoflavones. Thus, if you include soy or flaxseed in one of your meals every day, your intake will be roughly the same. Most of the recipes in this book that contain phytoestrogens have approximately that amount in a serving; many have much more.

Soy and hot flashes—the evidence. The effect of dietary soy supplementation on reducing hot flashes in menopausal women has recently been studied and published. In this study menopausal women requesting treatment for hot flashes were given 60 grams (about 2 ounces) of soy protein daily for 12 weeks. Soy was significantly superior to a placebo in reducing the number of hot flashes. By the end of the 12th week,

[7]H. Nagasawa. Nutrition and breast cancer: A survey of experimental and epidemiological evidence. *International Research Communications Journal of Medical Science* 8: 317–25, 1980.

[8]I. Kato, S. Tominaga, and T. Kuroishi. Relationship between westernization of dietary habits and mortality from breast and ovarian cancer in Japan. *Journal of Cancer Research and Clinical Oncology* 78: 349–57, 1987.

[9]D. P. Rose, A. P. Boyer, and E. L. Wynder. International comparison of mortality rates for cancer of the breast, ovary, prostate, and colon, per capita fat consumption. *Cancer* 58: 2363–71, 1986.

[10]D. M. Parkin. Cancers of the breast, endometrium and ovary: Geographical correlations. *European Journal of Cancer and Clinical Oncology* 25: 1917–25, 1989.

women taking soy had a 45 percent reduction in their daily hot flashes.[11]

Phytoestrogens and Their Protection against Breast and Other Cancers In some body structures phytoestrogens function as an antiestrogen and consequently have anticarcinogenic properties. Phytoestrogens bind to estrogen receptors in the body, but they do not elicit a large estrogenic response. Therefore, these phytoestrogens actually may prevent the body's estrogen from binding to receptors in some organ systems and could prevent estrogen-dependent cancers from forming. Breast, endometrial, and ovarian cancers are all stimulated by the presence of estrogen. Several studies have supported this protective effect of phytoestrogens in the development of these types of estrogen-dependent cancers.

In June 1990 the National Cancer Institute held a workshop to examine the relationship between soy in the diet and cancer prevention. The conclusions of this conference, based on epidemiological data,[12] indicated that soy consumption may lower colorectal cancer and that there is a moderate possibility that soy could help prevent breast cancer. More recent data from studies with animals[13] have confirmed a protective action against breast cancer.[14]

Soy and Heart Disease Prevention Studies also indicate that consumption of soy protein instead of animal protein, such as beef, decreases serum cholesterol concentrations. Soy is known

[11]P. Albertazzi, F. Pansini, and G. Bonaccorsi. The effect of dietary soy supplementation on hot flushes. *Obstetrics and Gynecology* 91: 6–11, 1998.

[12]D. P. Rose, A. P. Boyer, and E. L. Wynder. International comparison of mortality rates for cancer of the breast, ovary, prostate, and colon, per capita fat consumption. *Cancer* 58: 2363–71, 1986.

[13]S. Barnes, C. Grubbs, K. Setchell, et al. Soybeans inhibit mammary tumors in models of breast cancer. In Pariza, M., ed., *Mutagens and Carcinogens in the Diet* (New York: Wiley-Liss, 1990), pp. 239–53.

[14]C. A. Lamartiniere, J. B. Moore, N. M. Brown, et al. Genistein suppresses mammary cancer in rats. *Carcinogenesis* 16: 2833–40, 1995.

to lower cholesterol levels by 10 to 20 percent when one eats between 30 and 40 grams (1 to 1½ ounces) daily. A study published in 1995 in the *New England Journal of Medicine* indicates that an average daily consumption of 48 grams (1¾ ounces) of soy protein resulted in a 9.3 percent decrease in total cholesterol, a 12.9 percent decrease in LDL cholesterol, and a 10.5 percent decrease in triglyceride levels. These reductions are greater for those with moderate to severe hypercholesterolemia (>250 mg/dl).[15]

Cooking with Phytoestrogens Soy and other phytoestrogens are not typically a large part of the average American diet. However, these foods can be incorporated into meals with only minimal changes to more traditional cooking. They can be mixed with beef or other meats and incorporated into more traditional recipes. Tofu may be marinated and then will take on the flavor of the marinade. Silken tofu, a very creamy form of tofu, can be substituted for dairy products and oil in many recipes, making low-fat and phytoestrogen-rich cream sauces, salad dressings, and desserts.

Some soy products, such as vegetarian or soy burgers, are made with "soy-protein concentrate," which contains almost no isoflavones. These soy products do not have the phytoestrogen benefits of unprocessed soy products, such as tofu and miso. However, if you see "soy-protein isolate" on the label, the isoflavones largely are retained. So check the label carefully if you are eating some of the more "ready-made" soy products.

Phytoestrogens and Menopause—a Perfect Combination Phytoestrogens have been proven to decrease menopausal symptoms. Many women have turned to them as an alternative to hormone replacement therapy. Soy has been shown definitively to decrease heart disease, the number-one killer of

[15]J. W. Anderson, B. M. Johnston, and M. E. Newell. Meta-analysis of the effects of soy protein intake on serum lipids. *New England Journal of Medicine* 333: 276–82, 1995.

women, and this form of dietary estrogen actually may protect against breast and other cancers. While adding phytoestrogens to your daily diet may take some effort at first, it will be well worth the short-term benefits during menopause and the long-term benefits of a healthier life.

Chapter 3

Nutrition in Menopause

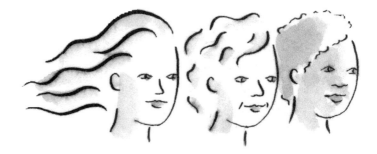

Understanding Your Diet

It is never too early or too late in life to start eating well. Because a woman's nutritional needs change after menopause, it is a good time to reevaluate your diet. Weight becomes more difficult to control and loss of calcium from bones accelerates, while iron loss from menstruation is no longer an issue. Most of these changes can be met by a simple, well-balanced diet that is low in fat and contains lots of fruits and vegetables.

The Dietary Guidelines Eating well can preserve your health, prevent disease, and increase your well-being. The most comprehensive advice comes from the Dietary Guidelines for Americans, published jointly by the U.S. Department of Agriculture and the U.S. Department of Health and Human Services. These guidelines were developed to help people obtain the nutrients they need, lead healthier, more active lives, and reduce their risk of certain chronic diseases.

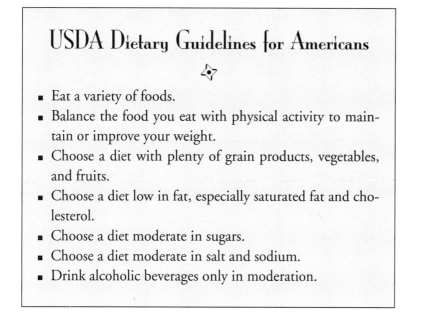

USDA Dietary Guidelines for Americans

- Eat a variety of foods.
- Balance the food you eat with physical activity to maintain or improve your weight.
- Choose a diet with plenty of grain products, vegetables, and fruits.
- Choose a diet low in fat, especially saturated fat and cholesterol.
- Choose a diet moderate in sugars.
- Choose a diet moderate in salt and sodium.
- Drink alcoholic beverages only in moderation.

Basic Components of the Diet Carbohydrates, protein, and fat are the basic components of your diet. The required amounts of those components are the same for women in menopause as for all adults. Therefore, you and your family can enjoy all of the meals in this book together.

For all individuals, at least half of your calories should come from carbohydrates, less than 30 percent of your calories should come from fat, and your protein sources should come from lean meats or vegetables. This means that your meals should be based upon foods like pasta, potatoes, grains, and fresh vegetables, with meat or other protein sources serving more as a garnish. The Chinese, among others, have known this for centuries.

Food Guide Pyramid The U.S. Department of Agriculture Food Guide Pyramid can be used to help you choose healthy foods in the correct proportions. The Food Guide Pyramid is a graphic representation of healthy eating; it replaces the basic four food groups that many of us learned in our youth. It symbolizes a balanced diet that arranges food into five groups to depict their proportion in your diet. For example, the bread, cereal, rice, and pasta group forms the base of the pyramid because most of the food you eat should come from that group.

The Food Guide Pyramid reinforces three concepts of healthful eating: balance, variety, and moderation. Your diet will be balanced when you eat more foods from the groups toward the base of the pyramid and fewer from food groups closer to the top. Variety means eating a variety of foods across and within each group in the pyramid.

The pyramid suggests a range of recommended daily servings from each food group—for example, three to five servings from the vegetable group. The lower number in each group is the recommended range for sedentary adults. The more active you are, the higher the number of servings you should eat from each food group.

Energy Sources

Carbohydrates Most of the calories in your diet should come from complex carbohydrates. This may come as a surprise since many think of menopause as a time when you should be limiting your intake of carbohydrates so that you do not gain too much weight. Many "quick weight loss" diets espouse very low carbohydrate diets. But carbohydrates should make up most of your diet in menopause and throughout your life because they are the preferred fuel for your body. Complex carbohydrates are broken down slowly by the body, especially if fiber is also present, providing a constant and steady energy source.

Carbohydrates come in two forms: simple carbohydrates,

Bread, Cereal, Rice, and Pasta Group

6–11 servings daily

A serving is:

   1 slice bread

   ½ bagel or English muffin

   1 ounce cold cereal

   ½ cup cooked cereal, rice, pasta, or grain

Vegetable Group

3–5 servings daily

A serving is:

   1 cup leafy greens or lettuce

   ½ cup cooked or raw vegetables

Fruit Group

2–4 servings daily

A serving is:

   1 medium apple, orange, pear, peach, or 1/2 banana

   ½ cup chopped, cooked, or canned fruit

   ¾ cup fruit juice

Milk, Yogurt, and Cheese Group

2–3 servings daily

A serving is:

   1 cup milk or yogurt

   1½ ounces cheese

   ½ cup part-skim ricotta cheese

   1 cup frozen yogurt

Meat, Poultry, Fish, Dry Beans, Eggs, and Nuts Group

2–3 servings daily

A serving is:

   2–3 ounces beef, poultry, or fish

   ½ cup cooked beans or legumes

   1 egg

   2 tablespoons peanut butter

Cheese

Eggs

Fish and shellfish

Lean meat

Milk

Poultry

Yogurt

Black beans

Bulgur

Chickpeas

Lentils

Miso

Pinto beans

Quinoa

Rice

Split peas

Tofu

White beans

which are found in fruits as well as sugar and candy, and complex carbohydrates, which are found in potatoes, vegetables, beans, and whole grains. Foods high in complex carbohydrates are also rich in important vitamins, minerals, and fiber. Fruits, although they contain simple sugars, are also a nutrient- and fiber-packed source of carbohydrates. Other simple-carbohydrate foods, such as candy and cookies, are full of "empty" calories since they generally contain few nutrients. (Diabetics may need to limit their intake of fruits and other simple carbohydrates.)

Protein The amount of protein recommended for your diet in menopause is 50 grams per day, the same as during other phases of your life cycle. That is not a large amount of protein: 10 grams of protein are found in 1 ounce of chicken or 1/3 cup of yogurt. The average American eats much more protein than is needed—on average, from 75 to 110 grams per day. Vegetarians will need more protein if it all comes from vegetable sources. But a vegetarian diet is perfectly adequate and can be very healthy for menopause, since vegetarian sources of protein are often lower in saturated fat.

While you generally will have no problem in filling your protein requirement during menopause, you should try to obtain protein from low-fat sources. Many people mistakenly believe that protein comes only from animal foods and dairy products, which may also contain undesirable amounts of fat and cholesterol. Yet foods such as grains and vegetables also contain protein.

Tofu and miso are excellent soy-based forms of protein, rich in both phytoestrogens and calcium, a perfect menopause protein source. Consuming several generous servings of these plant foods each day can help you meet a substantial portion of your protein requirement without increasing your intake of fat or cholesterol.

Fat Most health organizations, including the Food and Drug Administration (FDA) in its latest guidelines, recommend a diet that provides no more than 30 percent of calories from fat for all adults, including menopausal women. Some experts recommend keeping fat as low as 20 percent of your daily calories. However, the average American obtains more than 50 percent of his or her daily calories from fat. A high-fat diet, high blood cholesterol, and the development of coronary heart disease, which is the number-one killer of women, are interrelated.

In order to keep your intake of fat to 30 percent or less of your daily calories, you will need to choose low-fat protein sources, cut back on added oil in cooking and fried foods, eat approximately half of your calories from carbohydrates, and generally be aware of the fat content of the foods you eat. Note that essentially all the recipes in this book derive 30 percent or fewer calories from fat.

Saturated and unsaturated fat. Not all fat is equal. Fat is classified as saturated and unsaturated. It is saturated fat in the diet that has been associated most closely with the development of coronary heart disease. Saturated means that chemical bonds are saturated by hydrogen; unsaturated fats have fewer bonds occupied by hydrogen. Animal fats, particularly those found in red meat and dairy products, are predominantly saturated, whereas vegetable fats are predominantly unsaturated. Saturated fats include fat from butter, cheese, whole milk, and meat.

It is more healthful to make the majority of fat you consume come from unsaturated sources, such as canola, corn, safflower, and sunflower oil. Olive oil is monounsaturated, which has been shown to have a cholesterol-lowering effect, and is also a good choice. Unsaturated fats (such as oils) are mostly liquid at room temperature, while saturated fats (such as butter) are usually solid at room temperature.

Hydrogenated fat and **trans** *fatty acids.* Other types of fat found in foods as a result of chemical processing are hydrogenated fats and *trans* fatty acids. Originally manufactured with claims that they were more healthful than saturated fats, these types of fats have been found to promote heart disease in a fashion similar to that of saturated fats. *Trans* fatty acids were manufactured to increase the solidity of liquid unsaturated fats, so that, for example, oil could be converted to a spread.

Some of the chemical bonds in unsaturated fats have hydrogen added in a process known as hydrogenation. This changes the physical state of fat from liquid to solid by changing some unsaturated bonds to saturated. Margarine is an example of a fat that has been hydrogenated in order to convert it from a liquid to a solid. In a similar process in the case of *trans* fatty acids, the position of the hydrogen bond is changed from its natural position, known as *cis*, to an unnatural position, known as *trans*.

Products containing hydrogenated fats and *trans* fatty acids, especially margarine, were promoted heavily as being more healthful than foods containing saturated fat. It was thought that they did not raise blood cholesterol in the same manner that saturated fats did. However, such claims never were substantiated. Concerns have arisen because consumption of these hydrogenated vegetable fats and *trans* fatty acids has been tracked closely in time with coronary heart disease. *Trans* fatty acids have been found to affect the way cholesterol is processed in the bloodstream in a manner that increases the risk of heart disease.

The composition of dietary fat, rather than simply the quantity in your diet, is also of importance. Some recent studies have shown that replacing saturated fats, hydrogenated fats, and *trans* fatty acids with monounsaturated fats (such as olive oil) and unsaturated fats is more effective in preventing coronary heart disease in women than reducing overall fat intake. To be prudent, it is probably best to do both: Reduce your overall fat intake to less than 30 percent of your daily calories and make the majority of fat you consume unsaturated or olive oil.

Omega-3 fatty acids. One other type of fat is omega-3 fatty acids. These fats are from fish, especially fatty fish, such as salmon, swordfish, bluefish, mackerel, tuna, and wild striped bass. Such fats have been found to decrease the risk of coronary heart disease and thrombotic stroke. It is thought that they function as natural blood thinners, allowing the blood to flow more freely by not clogging the coronary arteries of the heart. You therefore should try to increase your intake of these types of fish in your diet.

Cholesterol

Cholesterol and Lipoproteins A high blood-cholesterol level (220 milligrams or more) is a well-established risk factor for coronary heart disease. Cholesterol, which is not a fat but a member of a chemical family called lipids, is very important in the body, forming the basic structure of many hormones, including estrogen.

Lipoproteins are complexes that carry fat in the bloodstream through the body. These complexes come in two major varieties: high-density lipoproteins (HDLs) and low-density lipoproteins (LDLs). Research has shown that high levels of HDLs (sometimes called the "good cholesterol"), which carry cholesterol to the liver for processing, are associated with a lower risk of heart disease. In contrast, high levels of LDLs (sometimes called the "bad cholesterol") are associated with a higher risk of heart disease. A high-cholesterol diet has been shown to lower HDLs, and raise LDLs, both of which are risk factors for developing heart disease. High levels of cholesterol in the blood, primarily cholesterol attached to LDL, are linked to an increased risk for coronary heart disease and heart attacks.

Blood-cholesterol levels. Most health-care providers advise trying to keep one's blood cholesterol less than 200 to 220 milligrams. Although cholesterol comes from your diet, it is also produced in the liver. Liver synthesis of cholesterol happens independently of dietary intake, but it is increased by the ingestion of saturated fats in the diet. To a degree, one's blood-cholesterol level is inherited, but diet can strongly affect it. The effect that dietary cholesterol has on blood cholesterol varies from person to person. For some people the amount of

Foods High in Cholesterol

Beef

Bacon

Butter

Cheese

Eggs

Whole milk

cholesterol in the diet has only a small effect on the level of cholesterol in the blood. But for others, especially people who already have high levels of blood cholesterol, dietary cholesterol can raise blood-cholesterol levels even further.

Diet and cholesterol. Your body makes most of the cholesterol circulating in your blood from the saturated fat you eat and, to a lesser degree, from the cholesterol in the food that you consume. Thus the two ways to keep your blood cholesterol low through dietary changes are to minimize your intake of foods high in saturated fats and cholesterol. Foods that are high in cholesterol are not necessarily high in fat or saturated fat, and vice versa. Vegetable oils, for example, are 100 percent fat but do not contain any cholesterol.

The best way to lower the overall fat, saturated fat, and cholesterol in your diet is to eat plenty of fruit, vegetables, and grains. Most of these foods in their natural form have little or no fat and are all cholesterol free. Certain foods are high in cholesterol and should be consumed in moderation: beef, bacon, butter, cheese, eggs, and whole milk.

A word about cholesterol in fish and shellfish: In general, fish and shellfish are low in fat and cholesterol, compared to beef, chicken, and dairy products. Although shellfish have a reputation for being high in cholesterol, this is not completely accurate. Shrimp, with about 150 milligrams of cholesterol in 3½ ounces, is now considered an acceptable alternative to red meat by the American Heart Association. Even lobster, which many on cholesterol-limited diets have been forbidden to eat, has only 70 to 95 milligrams of cholesterol per 3½ ounces. Compare an egg, with about 200 milligrams of cholesterol, or 3½ ounces of hamburger with 100 milligrams. The key here is, as always, moderation.

Preventing coronary heart disease. Your health-care provider may measure your blood lipid profile to determine your risk for developing coronary heart disease. High-cholesterol, low-HDL, and high-LDL levels are all risk factors for developing coronary heart disease. Your best defense against developing heart disease is to decrease your overall fat intake to 30 percent or fewer of your daily calories and consume mostly unsaturated or monounsaturated fat. In addition, consume as much omega-3–rich fish as you possibly can. These dietary measures, along with regular cardiovascular exercise, such as walking, jogging, or swimming, will do more to promote your heart health than any pill or medical intervention.

BETTER SOURCES OF FAT

Unsaturated fats	Monounsaturated fats	Omega-3 fatty acids
Canola oil	Olive oil	Anchovy
Corn oil		Bluefish
Sunflower oil		Mackerel
Safflower oil		Salmon
		Swordfish
		Wild striped bass
		Tuna

FATS TO TRY TO AVOID

Saturated fat	Hydrogenated fat	Cholesterol
Butter	Coconut oil	Beef
Beef	Margarine	Butter
Cheese	Palm oil	Cheese
Whole milk		Egg Yolk
		Liver
		Whole milk

Enriching Your Diet

Vitamins, Minerals, and Antioxidants Vitamin and mineral deficiencies are relatively uncommon in the United States. Most of us obtain enough vitamins and minerals from a well-balanced diet so that we do not need extra vitamins. The benefits of taking vitamin supplements in amounts that exceed the Recommended Dietary (or Daily) Allowance (RDA) remain uncertain.

Antioxidants include vitamin C, beta-carotene (which is converted to vitamin A in the body), and vitamin E. Research on the anticancer properties of antioxidants appears promising. What is still confusing is that antioxidants in the form of supplements may not have the same benefits as antioxidants when they are consumed in fruits and vegetables. Some studies have found that only when antioxidants are eaten in their natural state—in the form of fruits and vegetables, not when they are processed into vitamin supplements—do they exert their protective effect against a variety of cancers. Thus, your best defense is to be sure to eat a wide variety of both fruits and vegetables every day.

Calcium. Calcium is an important nutrient in menopause and deserves special mention. Calcium requirements in menopause are increased—1500 milligrams daily are currently recommended (1,000 milligrams daily for those taking hormone replacement therapy). Calcium is vital to the maintenance of strong bones. It also is involved on the cellular level in diverse body functions: the beating of your heart, controlling your blood pressure, and even in preventing premenstrual syndrome (something we hope you are finished with).

Achieving the recommended daily amounts of calcium is not difficult for people whose diets are rich in dairy products. Drinking three or four glasses of skim milk a day, for example, will get you close to your daily requirement through milk alone. But other sources of calcium, as well as calcium supplements, can provide a nondairy source.

Food is nearly always a better source of calcium than supplements, if for no other reason than food provides more nutritional benefits than calcium supplements and less risk of side effects. Dairy products are a well-known, rich source of calcium. In addition, tofu and certain vegetables are excellent nondairy calcium sources.

Dairy products. Milk is one of the best dietary sources of calcium for two reasons: the lactose, or milk sugar, that occurs naturally in milk and the vitamin D added to it enhance calcium absorption through the intestine. That process maximizes the amount of calcium your body obtains from each glass you drink. Because whole milk is also high in fat, I recommend that menopausal women drink skim milk, which retains all of the calcium content and almost none of the fat. I would choose skim over low-fat (2 percent) milk, since it has a fair amount of saturated fat, unless you really dislike the taste of skim milk. Most individuals find that once they switch to skim milk, after a few weeks they do not miss the flavor of whole or low-fat milk. In addition, choose nonfat over low-fat or whole-milk yogurt, as it is very similar in taste and texture, yet much healthier.

NUTRITIONAL COMPARISON OF WHOLE, LOW-FAT, AND SKIM MILK

1 cup	fat (grams)	calcium (mg)	calories (kcal)
whole milk	8.14	291	150
low-fat milk (2%)	4.78	297	121
skim milk	0.44	302	86

Dietary calcium is enhanced by vitamin D. But it is not generally necessary for all women to take vitamin D supplements. Being outside as little as 30 minutes a day in the sun will give your body ample amounts of this vitamin.

Weight Maintaining a healthy weight is one of the most important ways to prevent disease and maintain well-being. After menopause, weight control becomes more difficult, since metabolism begins to slow. I have no magic prescription for weight maintenance or loss in menopause. But following the basic guidelines of the Food Guide Pyramid and keeping the fat content of your diet low are the correct beginnings. Then the amount of calories you need to consume daily to maintain or lose weight depends upon your level of activity. The more active you are, the more you can eat. In my experience the one factor that ensures success in any weight maintenance or loss program is regular exercise. The best way to keep your weight under control for a lifetime is to maintain a healthy style of eating every day and not go on fad diets to lose weight quickly. Eating from the recipes in this book, which are all relatively low in fat and calories, is a good start.

Exercise Staying active is more important than ever before when you reach menopause. Even a small increase in your activity level can have a large effect on your overall health. You should get a total of 30 minutes of moderate exercise every day. Any type of activity counts toward that total—you do not necessarily need to join a gym or become an athlete. Daily activities such as yard work, gardening, and heavy cleaning are all beneficial. Exercise such as walking, jogging, swimming, playing tennis, and weight training are excellent physical activities during your entire life span. Staying fit and active will help you control your weight, increase your feelings of well-being, and help you sleep better. Remember, you can start out walking around the block and build up to longer, enjoyable walks or more physically strenuous exercise.

Chapter 4

Hormone Replacement Therapy: Yes or No?

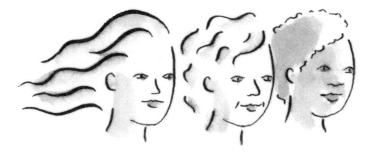

What Is Hormone Replacement Therapy?

Hormone Replacement Therapy (**HRT**) Hormone replacement therapy (HRT) is a medical intervention in which a woman takes medication containing estrogen and progesterone to replace the hormones her body is no longer producing. The long-term known health benefits of HRT that come from estrogen are increases in protection against heart disease and osteoporosis. However, taking estrogen alone (called unopposed estrogen) can cause the lining of the uterus to build up, increasing your chances of getting endometrial cancer, or cancer of the lining of the uterus. For protection from this, progesterone, which keeps the uterine lining from building up, is also given. In fact, women who take both estrogen and progesterone have a decreased incidence of endometrial cancer compared with those who do not take HRT at all. However, progesterone can decrease somewhat the health benefits of estrogen. Because its only purpose is to decrease the risk of endometrial cancer, women who have had a hysterectomy do not need to take it.

Varieties of Estrogen Supplements The most commonly prescribed estrogen supplements in the United States are conjugated equine estrogens, whose brand name is Premarin. Conjugated estrogens are derived from pregnant mares' urine. They are converted by the human body into an active form of estrogen. Other varieties of estrogen supplements are plant-based, with brand names such as Estrace, Estratab, Menest, Ogen, and Ortho-est. These forms have been marketed with claims of being more "natural" since they are produced from plants. They are converted into the same active forms of estrogen in your body as conjugated estrogens. To consider one form of estrogen more natural than another is not really relevant, since all of these estrogen supplements are produced in the lab. The only real difference is that one is animal-derived and the others are plant-derived. Estrogen supplements can be taken as pills, transdermal patches, and vaginal preparations. Pills have the advantage of being metabolized first by the liver, which enhances the beneficial effects of estrogen on cholesterol and lipids. Because the lipid-lowering effect is one of the major ways HRT prevents heart disease, I reserve transdermal patches and vaginal preparations for women who have side effects from oral preparations.

Estrogen comes in different dosages. Generally, the lowest dose is given—0.625 milligram for Premarin and 1 milligram for the plant-based estrogens—since that dose prevents osteoporosis and heart disease. However, sometimes newly menopausal women find that their symptoms of menopause, such as hot flashes, vaginal dryness, and mood changes, require a higher dose for full relief. After a year or two, the higher dosages usually can be lowered.

Varieties of Progesterone Supplements Several synthetic forms of progesterone, called progestogens, are available, the most commonly prescribed of which is medroxyprogesterone acetate (brand names Cycrin and Provera). Natural progesterone is not orally active; thus it must be altered in the lab into progestogens to retain its activity when taken orally. Recently, a new form of natural, orally active progesterone called micronized (broken down into small particles) progesterone has been developed. Synthetic progesterones tend to reduce estrogen's positive effect on cholesterol and lipids. The natural form of progesterone does not appear to do so. Thus, although both forms of progesterone are made in the lab, preliminary data indicate that the natural progesterone may be better for you.

Prescriptions of Hormone Replacement Therapy Two different methods for taking HRT are available: continuous or cyclic. Continuous means that you take both estrogen and progesterone every day. Because no cycling of the hormones occurs, you have no periods. In the cyclic method you take estrogen alone for part of the cycle and a combination of estrogen and progesterone for the rest of your cycle. Because of this, you will have a withdrawal bleeding, which is similar to having a period every month. The long-term health benefits of either method are the same. For women who prefer to have no further menses, the continuous method is preferable. For women who have trouble with breakthrough bleeding on continuous therapy or for those who find their side effects are fewer when progesterone is taken less often, the cyclic method is preferable.

Why Is Hormone Replacement Therapy Recommended?

Hormone Replacement Therapy for Relief of Menopausal Symptoms Women going through menopause often will have hot flashes, night sweats, and vaginal dryness because of the loss of estrogen in their bodies. The hot flashes and night sweats can cause sleep disturbances, making the women moody, irritable, and fatigued. HRT is an effective therapy for these problems. The duration of therapy for the treatment of menopausal symptoms varies but can range between a few months and a few years. In general, the younger the woman or the more abrupt the onset of the menopause, the worse these symptoms tend to be. The natural history of menopausal symptoms, without HRT, is that after a few months to a few years, they tend to decrease or go away entirely, except for vaginal dryness.

Hormone Replacement Therapy for Preventive Health
Hormone replacement therapy is effective in the prevention of osteoporosis and heart disease, both conditions for which postmenopausal women are at increased risk. Fractures from osteoporosis can have devastating effects on health and quality of life in older women. Many are surprised to know that heart disease, not cancer, is the number one killer of women. In addition, new evidence shows that the risk of Alzheimer's disease also may be reduced.

Hormone Replacement Therapy and Prevention of Osteoporosis HRT stabilizes bone-mineral density, and studies suggest that fracture risk is reduced between 30 percent and 50 percent for women taking HRT long-term (more than five years).[1] Estrogen is one of the drugs approved by the Food and Drug Administration for the prevention of osteoporosis. At risk for developing osteoporosis are women with a low body weight, Caucasian and Asian women, smokers, and women with a family history of osteoporosis. All women, regardless of risk, may benefit from diet and exercise to prevent osteoporosis. That

---

[1]J. A. Cauley, D. G. Seeley, K. Ensrud, et al. Estrogen replacement therapy and fractures in older women: Study of Osteoporotic Fractures Research Group. *Annals of Internal Medicine* 122: 9–16, 1995.

includes weight-bearing exercise—such as walking, running, aerobics, and weight training—and adequate calcium intake in the diet or in supplements. The current calcium recommendations are 1,500 milligrams a day for menopausal women not taking HRT and 1,000 milligrams a day for those taking HRT.

Hormone Replacement Therapy and Prevention of Heart Disease Heart disease is the most common cause of death among postmenopausal women. Studies have found a reduced rate of death from coronary heart disease (hardening of the arteries that supply the heart) among women who have taken HRT.[2] Estrogen causes the liver to produce more of the good cholesterol, HDL, and less of the bad cholesterol, LDL. Estrogen also inhibits the formation of artery-clogging plaque in the coronary arteries. The result of this improved lipid profile and protective effect on the heart is that women taking hormone replacement therapy have at least a 50 percent decrease in their risk of developing coronary heart disease.[3]

All women are at risk for heart disease, since it is the number-one cause of death in postmenopausal women. Women with personal risk factors for developing heart disease are those who are overweight, smoke, have high cholesterol, high blood pressure, or a family history of heart disease. All women, but particularly those in these risk groups, should discuss the pros and cons of HRT with their health-care providers.

Hormone Replacement Therapy and Prevention of Alzheimer's Disease A number of studies have suggested that women who take HRT may be at lower risk of developing

[2]D. Grady, S. M. Rubin, D. B. Petitti, et al. Hormone therapy to prevent disease and prolong life in postmenopausal women. *Annals of Internal Medicine* 117: 1016–37, 1992.

[3]M. J. Stampfer, W. C. Willett, G. A. Colditz, et al. A prospective study of postmenopausal estrogen therapy and coronary heart disease. *New England Journal of Medicine* 313: 1044, 1985.

Alzheimer's disease.[4] Supporting that possibility are studies in which women with Alzheimer's disease have demonstrated cognitive improvements after receiving estrogen.[5] Despite these exciting developments, many questions remain to be answered, and HRT should not be considered a proven preventive method for Alzheimer's disease.

When Is Hormone Replacement Therapy a Problem?

Side Effects of Hormone Replacement Therapy Side effects from HRT occur and persist in approximately 10 percent of women. The most frequent ones are bloating, nausea, mood changes, and breast tenderness. Women with migraine headaches may find that HRT precipitates the headaches. These side effects can be debilitating. Occasionally, changing the dosage of HRT or switching to different formulations can be helpful. Finally, for some women HRT is contraindicated for medical reasons. Women with a previous history of breast cancer or venous thrombosis should not take HRT. For these women, dietary interventions with phytoestrogens provide an alternative.

Hormone Replacement Therapy and Breast Cancer The fear of an increased risk of breast cancer is perhaps the principal reason women choose not to use hormone replacement therapy. Data on the effects of long-term hormone replace-

[4]M. X. Tang, D. Jacobs, Y. Stern, et al. Effect of oestrogen during menopause on risk and age at onset of Alzheimer's disease. *Lancet* 348: 429–32, 1996.

[5]V. W. Henderson, A. Paganini-Hill, C. K. Emanuel, et al. Estrogen replacement therapy in older women: Comparisons between Alzheimer's disease cases and nondemented control subjects. *Archives of Neurology* 51: 896–900, 1994.

ment therapy on the risk of developing breast cancer[6] have demonstrated an increased risk in women taking these drugs. Women who used hormones 10 or more years are approximately 150 percent as likely to develop breast cancer as those who do not take hormones. For women with a strong family history of breast cancer, such as it occurring in two first-degree relatives (mother or sister) or having a mother who died of breast cancer at a premenopausal age, the risk may be higher. This has reinforced fears and reservations that many women and their physicians have about this form of treatment.

Raloxifen: A New Estrogen Raloxifen is the newest addition to a woman's choice of menopausal therapies. Raloxifen is a synthetic preparation made in the laboratory of a type of estrogen that acts on some parts of the body but not on others, a so-called *selective estrogen receptor modulator*. For example, Raloxifen is active on bones and lipids and has been shown to prevent osteoporosis and heart disease in the same fashion as traditional hormone replacement therapy. However, studies have been going on in this country for only up to three years, so it is not as well proven. Raloxifen is not active on the breast, so it has the additional benefit of not increasing a woman's risk of breast cancer; some preliminary evidence suggests that it may even decrease a woman's breast cancer risk. However, it does not prevent hot flashes and resulting sleep disturbances, so it is not generally advised for newly menopausal women with those symptoms. It is not active on the vaginal tissues, so it will not improve vaginal dryness. Thus, for long-term health benefits, Raloxifen is a promising alternative to HRT. However, for the short-term discomforts of menopause—hot flashes, resulting sleep disturbances, and vaginal dryness—Raloxifen does not help. Again, even if you are taking Raloxifen, it is still important to eat a proper diet and exercise.

[6]G. A. Colditz, S. E. Hankinson, D. J. Hunter, et al. The use of estrogen and progestin and the risk of breast cancer in postmenopausal women. *New England Journal of Medicine* 332: 1589–93, 1995.

Medicalization of Menopause Many women feel strongly that since menopause is a natural phase of the life cycle, they do not wish to have it medicalized by taking hormones. Currently, only 15 percent of women who are eligible for hormone replacement therapy are using it. Thus, a major need exists for offering alternatives to hormone replacement therapy in order to maintain health and wellness during menopause.

A Woman's Decision

To Take or Not to Take Women, with the help of their medical providers, must consider carefully the pros and cons for their particular situation in deciding whether to take hormone replacement therapy. For example, women with a personal or family history of heart disease or osteoporosis may benefit greatly from hormone replacement therapy and feel those benefits outweigh any other risks. On the other hand, women with a strong family history of breast cancer, such as women with two first-degree relatives or a mother who died of breast cancer at a premenopausal age, may not want to further increase their risk of getting breast cancer. These women should seek alternative therapies for menopausal symptoms, heart disease, and osteoporosis prevention, including diet.

Individual Choices Women experience menopause as individuals, and generalizations cannot be made about what is the best way for each woman to care for herself in menopause. Women become menopausal in a variety of ways. Some women begin menopause as young as their 30s or 40s, while others start as late as their 60s. The average age of menopause is 52. Women who undergo a premature menopause—menopause under the age of 40—should strongly consider some type of hormone replacement therapy. Women have varying degrees of menopausal symptoms and different family risk factors for diseases that are affected by estrogen. If you are taking HRT only for the short-term relief of menopausal symptoms, you will likely need them only for a year or two. However, it you are taking HRT for the long-term health benefits, you will take them for the rest of your life. While the benefits will not go away entirely if you stop taking them, they are maximized if you continue them throughout your life.

Diet, Exercise, and Preventive Health All women, whether or not they take HRT, should eat a diet low in saturated fat and cholesterol and rich in calcium, fruits, and vegetables. Fat should be kept to less than 30 percent of your daily calories. Soy, in the form of tofu, miso, and soy milk has been shown to have protective effects on coronary heart disease, and it should be incorporated into your diet. Cardiovascular exercise should be incorporated into your daily routines. You should aim to do some type of cardiovascular exercise—walking, jogging, aerobics, bicycling—for 25 to 30 minutes a minimum of three days per week. These lifestyle interventions should be incorporated whether or not you decide to use hormone replacement therapy.

Chapter 5

Preventing Osteoporosis

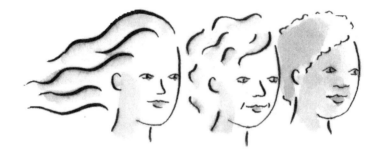

What Is Osteoporosis?

Osteoporosis is a disease in which the skeleton thins, causing the bones to become fragile and leading to an increased risk of bone fractures. It has no symptoms until a fracture occurs many years later. Osteoporosis affects 25 million Americans, mostly women. It becomes much more common after a woman goes through menopause, because estrogen protects her bones before this time.

Bones and Calcium Regulation in the Body In order to understand how osteoporosis affects the bones, it is necessary to understand the relationship of bones and the regulation of calcium in the body. Bones consists of a matrix of collagen containing calcium and phosphate. The most significant function of bone is actually not as a supporting structure, but rather as a calcium reservoir for many body functions. Calcium is an essential element for all cell functions. The heart requires calcium to beat, the muscles require calcium to function, and the nervous system requires calcium to transmit messages. We must eat calcium-rich foods to supply these needs, and a reserve supply of calcium is stored in bones. For normal cellular activity, blood-calcium levels must be maintained in a very tight range. The reservoir of calcium in the skeleton is critical in allowing a steady supply of calcium for cellular functions at a moment's notice.

Osteoblasts and Osteoclasts Osteoblasts are cells in the body that function to resorb bone and release calcium into the bloodstream. Another related cell, the osteoclast, acts exactly opposite to the osteoblast by forming new bone. Normally, the actions of osteoblasts and osteoclasts balance each other so that bone density is maintained during the process of calcium metabolism. Estrogen appears to decrease bone resorption by inhibiting the action of osteoblasts. Thus, when estrogen levels are decreased after menopause, more bone is resorbed because the osteoblasts are disinhibited—that is, the osteoblasts have freer range in the body to resorb bone. Resorption of bone by osteoblasts causes the bones to become less dense, and once the decreased density reaches a critical level, bones are susceptible to fractures.

The good news is that osteoporosis is preventable and treatable. Bone health is influenced by three major interacting factors: diet, exercise, and estrogen. Good nutrition, for example, is estimated to decrease its incidence by one-half. Your best defense against osteoporosis is prevention.

How Bones Form in Your Premenopausal Years Your ultimate bone density is partially predetermined by your genetics, but it can also be affected by other factors. Early lifestyle affects your ultimate peak bone mass, which is reached somewhere between ages 30 and 35. Most of your bone density, though, is achieved by about age 20, the time at which you've stopped growing. Premenopausally, while your bones are growing, calcium and exercise make them stronger and denser. Alcohol intake and cigarette smoking lower your bone mass.

Only while bones still are growing can they be made denser. That small window of opportunity in increasing the bone density in girls and women has only recently been recognized, and this recognition emphasizes the importance of diet, exercise, and avoidance of smoking in young women. After this time bones cannot be made denser by diet, calcium, lifestyle, or hormones. All later interventions can only prevent further bone loss. Some experts predict an epidemic of osteoporosis in future years because today's children and teenagers are consuming only about half the amount of calcium from foods that young people did in 1950.

Risk Factors for Osteoporosis Bone mass is more dense in African American, overweight, active, and tall women and less dense in short, frail, thin-skinned, sedentary women. Thus, women in the former group usually do not develop osteoporosis, whereas women in the latter group are at greater risk for developing the disorder and may lose bone mass gradually and continually each year after menopause.

Menopause and Osteoporosis After menopause, if you do not use preventive measures, you lose bone at an average rate of approximately 5 percent per year. By the end of only five years, that loss can deplete your bone mass to extremely low levels. Fractures start to occur when you have bone loss of around 35 to 50 percent. At that point it is almost impossible to reverse this loss. Stopping bone loss at an earlier stage prevents bone density from falling below that fracture threshold.

Mechanism of Bone Loss Menopausal bone loss results from estrogen deficiency. Bone loss is mainly due to an increase in

Risk Factors for Osteoporosis

✧

- Cigarette smoking
- Early menopause
- Endocrine disorders, such as diabetes mellitus, hyperthyroidism, and Cushing's disease
- Family history of osteoporosis
- High caffeine intake
- High alcohol intake
- High protein intake
- Low calcium intake
- Low vitamin D intake
- Low weight in relation to height
- Race: Caucasian or Asian
- Sedentary lifestyle

resorption of bone by osteoblasts. Human osteoblasts normally eat away at bone in order to maintain calcium levels in your bloodstream. Bone loss normally is counteracted by the actions of osteoclasts, which lay down new bone. This dynamic process allows calcium to be released into the bloodstream, yet maintains the skeleton. After menopause the homeostasis can be lost. Osteoblasts appear to have estrogen receptors, and when estrogen is low, they become more active in resorbing bone. Estrogen increases the levels of the hormone calcitonin, which also acts to prevent bone resorption. Therefore, there may be several mechanisms whereby estrogen prevents bone loss.

Diagnosis of Osteoporosis Bone density measurements are tests that may be used to determine the risk of developing osteoporosis. At least 25 percent of bone needs to be lost before osteoporosis is diagnosed by routine X-ray examination. A bone density study can be performed before that amount of loss to determine whether your bones are thinning.

Bone density can be measured by a number of different techniques. At present dual energy X-ray absorptiometry (DXA) is the most commonly utilized method. DXA can be used both for assessments of risk and in serial measurements as a follow-up to assess therapy results.

Not all women need a bone density study. Bone-mineral density measurements are not routinely necessary unless the information gained will be useful in helping you to make decisions about starting therapy. Indications for a bone density study include a personal history of two risk factors for osteoporosis (see list on page 59) or a decision at menopause not to take hormone replacement therapy. If bones are found to be below the average density—less than two standard deviations below the mean value for healthy young women— therapy is recommended to prevent the development of osteoporosis.

If you are determined to be at risk for osteoporosis based upon bone density testing, you usually have time to institute some preventive or treatment measures before fractures occur. Some women and their health-care providers find bone-mineral density measurements helpful in making their own personal decisions about whether to begin hormonal therapy.

Fractures from Osteoporosis The most common places fractures occur as a result of osteoporosis are in the spine, hip, and wrist, but they can occur in almost any bone in the body. Currently, those three major osteoporosis types of fracture represent more than 1.5 million fractures each year in the United States.[1] By age 80, 20 percent of all Caucasian women will develop hip fractures, and about 15 percent will die from the fracture itself or from complications within 6 months. About 15,000 women die of osteoporosis or its complications annually in the United States, and hip fractures are the twelfth lead-

[1]L. J. Melton III, A. W. Lane, C. Cooper, et al. Prevalence and incidence of vertebral deformities. *Osteoporosis International* 3: 113–19, 1993.

ing cause of death in women in the United States. As the population ages, this problem will continue to escalate.

Therapies to Prevent Bone Loss

Strategies to prevent and treat osteoporosis include dietary changes, calcium supplementation, exercise, and hormone or other drug therapies. Regardless of whether you are taking hormones or other drugs, you can benefit from a diet rich in calcium and from regular exercise.

Calcium and Prevention of Bone Loss The recommended daily allowance for calcium for menopausal women is currently 1,500 milligrams daily or 1,000 milligrams for women taking hormone replacement therapy. Adequate dietary calcium and calcium supplementation postmenopausally does not completely arrest bone loss but will slow it by 30 to 50 percent. The full amount of calcium may be incorporated into a healthy diet, but it does require paying attention to the calcium content of the foods you eat.

Calcium is found in good quantities in dairy products and some dark green leafy vegetables. It is difficult, but not impossible, to meet calcium requirements without consuming dairy products. Those who do consume dairy products will find they can meet the requirement with relative ease. It is important to watch which dairy products you eat, since many of them, in addition to being good sources of calcium, are unfortunately very high in fat. For high-calcium alternatives to milk products, also eat greens from the cole family: kale, collards, broccoli, and bok choy.

Some substances can hinder the absorption of calcium, including oxalic acid (found in spinach and Swiss chard) and phytic acid (found in tea and the outer layers of whole grains). These substances form insoluble compounds with calcium, binding it in such a way that it cannot be absorbed from the intestine. Therefore, you may not absorb as much calcium in foods containing them.

Food	Quantity	Calcium (mg)
Dairy products		
Blue cheese	1 ounce	183
Frozen yogurt	½ cup	147
Ice cream, soft vanilla	1 cup	236
Mozzarella	1 ounce	147
Milk, whole	1 cup	291
Milk, skim	1 cup	302
Parmesan	1 ounce	336
Ricotta, part skim	½ cup	337
Romano	1 ounce	330
Yogurt, nonfat	1 cup	415
Beans and legumes		
Black beans	½ cup cooked	30
Chickpeas	½ cup cooked	45
Soybeans	½ cup cooked	131
Soybeans, dry roasted	½ cup	232
Soy milk	1 cup	46
Tempeh	2 ounce	47
Tofu	2 ounce	154
Vegetables and fruits		
Bok choy	1 cup	116
Broccoli, cooked	1 cup	132
Collard greens	1 cup	357
Dandelion greens	1 cup	147
Fortified juices	1 cup	300
Kale	1 cup	206
Mustard greens	1 cup	193
Romaine lettuce	1 cup	37
Sea vegetables (wakame)	¼ cup dry	67
Spinach	1 cup	56
Swiss chard	1 cup	128
Turnip greens	1 cup	252

Nuts and seeds

Almonds	2 tbs	42
Pine nuts	1 ounce	38
Sesame seeds	2 tsp	218
Tahini	2 tbs	139

Calcium supplements. For those who do not eat any dairy products or are lactose intolerant, it is difficult but not impossible to obtain from your diet the necessary amount of calcium your body requires. You may find it necessary to supplement your diet with calcium supplements. If you are not obtaining adequate calcium from your diet, I recommend taking a daily calcium supplement containing approximately 1,000 milligrams. Calcium supplements are sold over the counter and come in many forms. It does not make much difference which type you choose in order to meet your daily requirement of calcium; calcium supplements in many forms are absorbed in a similar fashion by the body. There are some tricks to maximizing your absorption of calcium from supplements. They are best absorbed when taken with meals, and small doses at a time are better absorbed than one large dose.

Women taking hormone replacement therapy should be aware that maintaining good calcium intake yields benefits above and beyond those conferred by the hormones on their bones. Calcium has been shown in numerous studies to aid in the prevention of colon cancer. Adequate dietary calcium can prevent some types of hypertension (high blood pressure). So even if you are taking hormone replacement therapy, you should take measures to ensure the calcium content of your diet.

Exercise and Prevention of Osteoporosis Many studies have demonstrated that exercise increases bone density. The best exercises for increasing bone density are those that are weight-bearing. Jogging, aerobics, walking, strength training, and tennis are examples of weight-bearing exercise. Swimming, by contrast, is not a weight-bearing exercise. Benefits of strength training have been shown from as little as two days of exercise per week. In general, it is best to aim for 30 minutes of exercise performed three days per week.

The gains that postmenopausal women make by vigorous, weight-bearing exercise must be maintained by continued exercise, or the bones will revert over a very short time to their pre-exercise state. Thus, exercise must be continued for a lifetime to protect your bones. In addition to increasing bone density, exercise also promotes better balance and strength, which decreases the number of falls and fractures, especially in the elderly.[2] Recent studies suggest that this effect of better balance and strength actually may be the more important factor in the beneficial effects of exercise in decreasing the incidence of fractures[3]. It is becoming evident that strength training is particularly beneficial in this fashion.

Estrogen Replacement and Other Drugs for Prevention of Bone Loss There is no question that hormones affect bone mass. Premenopausally, pregnancy and the use of oral contraceptives increase bone density. Women who do not ovulate regularly and have low estrogen levels, such as some athletes and women of low body weight, have an increased risk for osteoporosis later in life. Postmenopausally, many studies have shown that estrogen therapy reduces the amount of bone loss as well as the incidence of fractures.[4] When hormones are stopped, the bone loss resumes.[5]

[2]M. A. Province, E. C. Hadley, M. C. Hornbrook, et al. The effects of exercise on falls in elderly patients: A preplanned meta-analysis of the FIC-SIT trials. *Journal of the American Medical Association* 273: 1341–47, 1995.

[3]M. E. Nelson, M. A. Fiatorone, C. M. Morganti, et al. Effects of high-intensity strength training on multiple risk factors for osteoporotic fractures. A randomized controlled trial. *Journal of the American Medical Association* 272: 1909–14, 1994.

[4]N. S. Weiss, C. L. Ure, J. H. Ballard, et al. Decreased risk of fractures of the hip and lower forearm with postmenopausal use of estrogen. *New England Journal of Medicine* 303: 1195, 1980.

[5]B. Ettinger, H. K. Genant, and C. E. Cann: Long-term estrogen replacement therapy prevents bone loss and fractures. *Annals of Internal Medicine* 102: 319, 1985.

Drugs used for the prevention and treatment of osteoporosis fall into several major classes. Hormone replacement therapy is indicated for the prevention and treatment of osteoporosis. It is the most common therapy for preventing or limiting the bone loss that occurs in women after menopause. Although the precise mechanism whereby estrogen prevents a decrease in bone density is not known, human osteoblast cells have estrogen receptors, and it is likely that estrogen therapy decreases bone loss by acting directly on those receptors. Estrogen also increases calcitonin levels, and calcitonin prevents bone resorption. In one study women taking HRT experienced 35 percent fewer hip fractures than those not taking HRT. HRT has the added advantage of preventing heart disease, the main cause of death in women. However, HRT may increase one's risk of breast cancer and can have bothersome side effects, such as bleeding, breast tenderness, bloating, and mood swings.

Selective estrogen receptor modulators (SERMs) are a new type of estrogen that acts on some specific sites in the body, such as bones and the cardiovascular system, as an estrogen, but as an antiestrogen in others, such as the breast and uterus. Raloxifen (Evista) is a SERM that is indicated for the prevention of osteoporosis. Raloxifen can be taken at any time of the day, with or without food. Raloxifen appears to prevent fractures almost as well as traditional HRT. Side effects are few but include hot flashes and leg cramps.

Antiresorptive agents are a class of drugs that both prevent and treat osteoporosis by inhibiting osteoclast-mediated bone resorption. Alendronate (Fosamax) is the most widely studied. It needs to be taken at least a half hour before any other food or pills with a 6- to 8-ounce glass of water. Taking it with other liquids, foods, or medications will decrease its absorption and lessen its effectiveness. Because of its potential for esophageal irritation, one should not lie down for a half hour after taking Alendronate. For the same reason it should not be taken before bedtime. Alendronate can decrease fracture rates by as much as 50 percent in high-risk populations. Calcitonin is another antiresorptive agent. The hormone, which is synthesized in the thyroid, works by inhibiting the cells that eat bone, the osteoclasts. It currently is used only for treatment of osteoporosis, not prevention. It is not active orally and must be taken either by injection or intra-nasal spray. Current studies regarding its effectiveness are ongoing.

Summary Preventing osteoporosis is best started in childhood, since that is the time when bones still are growing and therefore have the potential to increase their calcium content. It is important that children and young women eat a diet rich in calcium and get regular exercise. For menopausal women the goal is to prevent bone loss in order to maintain the density of the bones that has been previously obtained, since it no longer is possible to increase bone density at this time. Such prevention is best achieved through a combination of a diet rich in calcium and regular weight-bearing exercise. Hormones or other drugs can be added to these measures for those individuals found to be at significant risk for osteoporosis.

Chapter 6

Preventing Heart Disease

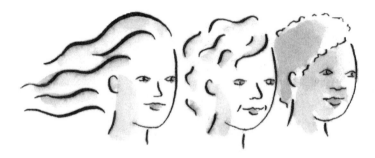

Menopause and Coronary Disease

Arteriosclerosis, hardening of the coronary arteries of the heart, is the most common cause of death in women. Coronary artery disease becomes much more common after menopause, since the estrogen produced by the body before this time has a protective effect on the heart. Women are less resistant to coronary disease after menopause.[1] While arte-

[1] K. A. Matthews, R. R. Wing, L. H. Kuller, et al. Influence of the peri-menopause on cardiovascular risk factors and symptoms of middle-aged healthy women. *Archives of Internal Medicine* 154: 2349–55, 1994.

riosclerosis is common, it is also preventable. A diet low in fat, a regular exercise routine, and replacement of the estrogen your body now lacks will prevent heart disease for most women.

Heart Disease in Women and Men Under the age of 50, men have a much greater incidence of heart attacks caused by arteriosclerosis—hardening of the arteries of the heart—than women. In both sexes the incidence increases as we age. But after 50 in women, the rate of heart attacks increases, and by age 80 it is equal to that of men. Studies have shown that taking estrogen during menopause delays the development of arteriosclerosis in postmenopausal women[2] and reduces the risk of developing a heart attack or dying from a heart attack.[3]

Women versus men. Heart disease in women is different from that in men. The first symptom of coronary heart disease in women is likely to be angina (chest pain), whereas in men it is more likely to be a heart attack. Death, however, from cardiovascular disease is actually more common in women than in men. The reason is that nearly two-thirds of sudden deaths caused by heart attacks in women occur in those with no previous symptoms of disease, compared with about half the sudden deaths in men. Treatment for heart disease in women may be less likely to be effective in reducing the death rate because the majority of women never may reach a hospital. For those women primary prevention is likely to be the only solution. Heart disease in men has received a great deal of attention, but this important problem in women needs to be addressed equally.

Lipid Changes in Menopause After menopause, estrogen deficiency leads to higher LDL cholesterol (bad cholesterol) and lower HDL cholesterol (good cholesterol). The overall effect is a more unfavorable lipid profile that is thought to contribute to the development of atherosclerosis, or hardening of the arteries.

[2]J. M. Sullivan, R. Vander Zwaag, J. P. Hughes, et al. Estrogen replacement and coronary artery disease. *Archives of Internal Medicine* 150: 2557, 1990.

[3]D. B. E. Henderson, A. Paganini-Hill, and R. K. Ross. Decreased mortality in users of estrogen replacement therapy. *Archives of Internal Medicine* 151: 75, 1991.

Blood Vessel Changes in Menopause In addition to the lipid changes, estrogen has a direct effect on blood vessel walls. Estrogen promotes relaxation of blood vessel walls, allowing them to remain open and reducing their clogging by arteriosclerosis. After menopause, with estrogen levels lowered, that relaxation effect is lost.

Decreasing Coronary Risk

Preventive Strategies Efforts to prevent or retard the progression of cardiovascular disease in women should focus on a woman's total cardiovascular risk profile. In addition to some form of estrogen replacement (phytoestrogens or hormone replacement therapy) a heart-healthy plan includes exercise, weight control, a low-fat diet, cholesterol control, blood pressure control, and no smoking. These lifestyle interventions are very effective in preventing heart disease.

Soy and heart disease prevention. Several studies have documented that replacing animal protein in the diet with soy protein has a cholesterol-lowering effect. This effect is particularly evident in those with inherited tendencies for high blood-cholesterol levels. Thus, one dietary change that you can make toward preventing heart disease is to replace some of the meat in your diet with tofu and miso.

Hormone replacement therapy and heart disease. Numerous studies have found a reduced rate of mortality from coronary heart disease among women who have taken hormone replacement therapy.[4] The mechanisms by which estrogen favorably influences cardiovascular risk factors are many. Hormone replacement therapy, similar to the body's natural estrogen, affects the production of lipoproteins in the liver, producing more of the good cholesterol, HDL, and less of the bad cholesterol, LDL. Hormone replace-

[4]D. Grady, S. M. Rubin, D. B. Petitti, et al. Hormone therapy to prevent disease and prolong life in postmenopausal women. *Annals of Internal Medicine* 117: 1016–37, 1992.

ment therapy also directly inhibits plaque formation in the coronary arteries and enhances substances that dilate the coronary arteries, preventing them from getting clogged.

Exercise. Advice about preventing heart disease would not be complete without some mention of exercise. Exercise increases your sense of well-being, helps control your weight, and improves the health of your heart. Life for most of us has become increasingly complex and busy. But exercise can and must be incorporated into your lifestyle. My advice to busy individuals is to incorporate exercise into your daily routines: walk to work, to the train, during your lunch hour, or to stores when you run your errands; join a fitness center that you can visit during lunchtime or just before or after work; purchase good-quality exercise machines for your home, such as a stationary bicycle or treadmill. You should aim to accumulate 30 minutes of moderately intense physical activity daily, a minimum of three times per week.

Risk Factors for Heart Disease

Blood pressure. Many studies have shown an association between elevated blood pressure and risk of coronary heart disease and stroke in both women and men. Studies also have shown that controlling blood pressure through weight reduction and antihypertensive (blood pressure lowering) medication results in a significant reduction in the development of coronary heart disease and stroke. Regular checkups with your health-care provider are important so that elevated blood pressure can be screened, since it generally has no symptoms.

Smoking. Cigarette smoking remains the leading preventable cause of coronary heart disease in women, with more than 50 percent of heart attacks among middle-aged women attributable to tobacco.[5] The risk of developing heart disease

[5]W. C. Willett, A. Green, M. J. Stampfer, et al. Relative and absolute excess risks of coronary heart disease among women who smoke cigarettes. *New England Journal of Medicine* 317: 1303–9, 1987.

begins to decline within months of quitting smoking and reaches the level of those who have never smoked within 3 to 5 years. While quitting smoking is no easy task, studies have shown that the more times you attempt to quit, the more likely your next try will be successful. Speak to your healthcare provider about setting a date for quitting, obtaining nicotine substitutes, utilizing hypnosis, and joining group therapy. One of these methods might work for you.

Alcohol. Moderate amounts of alcohol (one to two drinks per day) may provide some protection from coronary heart disease. However, higher amounts of alcohol have the opposite effect, causing alcohol-related heart disease. In addition, alcohol consumption is linked to several types of cancers, including breast cancer, with intake as little as 2 drinks per day. Thus, you should limit yourself to 1 to 2 drinks per day.

Stress. Mental stress, type-A personalities, and job stress all have been linked with the development of coronary heart disease. Recent studies on the effects of relaxation techniques and lifestyle changes that reduce stress show great promise. As a holistic approach to menopausal health, reduce stress by simplifying your life as much as possible and learn relaxation techniques to better handle the stresses that remain.

Preventing Heart Disease The prevention of heart disease can become a part of every woman's healthy lifestyle. You should eat a low-fat and phytoestrogen-rich diet. You should perform cardiovascular exercise at least three times a week. Keep your blood pressure controlled, do not smoke, use alcohol in moderation, and keep stress to a minimum. You will find life enjoyable, your energy high, and personal fulfillment maximized by these important interventions.

Chapter 7

Cancer Prevention

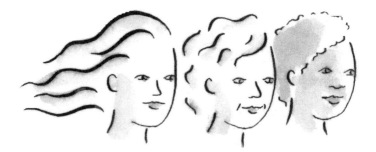

Cancer, especially breast cancer, is every woman's greatest fear. Fortunately, you can take measures to prevent breast and other cancers. Dietary adjustments, exercise, and avoidance of such things as smoking and excessive alcohol can prevent many types of cancer. Those simple measures are far more effective than worrying about eating organic foods, drinking bottled water, or avoiding environmental exposures, and they are things you can directly control. You do not need to live in a bubble to greatly decrease your chances of getting cancer. Of course, many cancer cases still develop despite the best health-promoting behavior.

Dietary adjustments are a particularly powerful way to practice cancer prevention while promoting overall good health and well-being. Soy in the diet has been shown to decrease the risk of breast cancer effectively. Antioxidants from vitamins found in fruits and vegetables lower the incidence of a whole variety of cancers. Fiber and calcium in the diet aid in the prevention of colon cancer. A diet low in saturated fat helps prevent colon, rectal, and possibly breast cancer. Maintaining your optimal body weight decreases your risk of colon and breast cancer.

Breast Cancer

Breast cancer is the most frequently diagnosed malignancy in women today. American women have a lifetime probability of developing breast cancer of 12.2 percent, about one in eight.[1] The incidence of breast cancer has been increasing steadily throughout the world. This increase has received a great deal of publicity, and many women live in fear of developing the disease. But you can take measures to prevent the development of breast cancer.

Risks for Breast Cancer Any woman is at risk for developing breast cancer. Known risk factors, such as older age, early menarche (age of onset of periods), no children or late age of first pregnancy, late menopause, family history of breast cancer, and obesity, account for only 40 to 50 percent of breast cancer cases. Consequently, 50 to 60 percent of cases have causes that are unknown. Thus, all women should take measures to prevent breast cancer.

Nutrition and Prevention of Breast Cancer Perhaps no area is more controversial than the link between nutrition and breast cancer, in particular, the association between dietary fat and the development of breast cancer. Findings from animal research suggest that saturated fat in the diet may play a role in the development of breast cancer. But studies in humans are conflicting,

[1]Cancer facts and figures. American Cancer Society, 1994.

with earlier studies finding this same association, but more recent and well controlled studies not confirming it. These studies show no evidence of an association of saturated fat intake with any increased risk of developing breast cancer. In reviewing the data on thousands of women from six major research studies on women's health—California Seventh-Day Adventists Study, Nurses' Health Study, Canadian Breast Cancer Screening Study, Iowa Women's Studies, New York State Cohort, and Dutch Cohort—no association was made with intake of saturated fat and the incidence of breast cancer. When comparing pre- and postmenopausal women, no stronger association was made with the older women and fat intake and breast cancer. Finally, the studies did not indicate that keeping calories from fat to 30 percent or less of total calories reduces the incidence of breast cancer, as has been suggested in the past.[2]

The medical literature offers some conflicting evidence about the protective effect of olive oil, which is monounsaturated, as well as unsaturated fats and the risk of breast cancer. Small studies present some evidence that these types of fats may protect against the development of breast cancer.[3] We do know that those same fats—and a low-fat diet—protect you from the development of heart disease. Given such conflicting data, it is prudent to keep the overall fat content in your diet to 30 percent or fewer of your daily calories, and that the majority of the fat you eat comes from olive oil (monounsaturated) or unsaturated fat sources. That approach is good for your overall health, so if it also protects you from breast cancer, all the more reason to continue it.

Antioxidants in the Diet Beta-carotene, vitamin A, and vitamin E are all antioxidants found in many fruits and vegetables that have been shown to have a protective effect against the

[2]W. C. Willett and D. J. Hunter. Prospective studies of diet and breast cancer. *Cancer* 74: 1085–89, 1994.

[3]S. Franceschi, A. Favero, A. Decarli, et al. Intake of macronutrients and risk of breast cancer. *Lancet* 347: 1351–56, 1996.

development of many cancers.[4] Antioxidants are chemicals that keep other substances from being oxidized. For example, when an apple is left out and turns brown, it is being oxidized. Vitamin C is a natural antioxidant that is used in cooking to prevent changes caused by oxidation, such as foods turning brown or rancid. When we sprinkle a cut apple with lemon or lime juice (which contains vitamin C) to keep it from turning brown, we're preventing oxidation. In the human body antioxidants have been shown to prevent cells from turning cancerous. In addition, antioxidants keep LDL from being oxidized. It is oxidized LDL that may be the true culprit behind arterial plaque buildup in atherosclerosis.

Beta-carotene, vitamin C, and vitamin E are all effective antioxidants. Recent medical studies indicate that antioxidants in the diet may prevent many types of cancer as well as heart disease caused by atherosclerosis. Scientific research has shown that antioxidant vitamins have their greatest protective effect when they are eaten as part of the diet, not as vitamin supplements. Several studies have shown that antioxidant vitamins have no cancer protection effect when they are taken only as vitamin supplements. Antioxidants may work in conjunction with other elements in the fruit or vegetable, so it is best to consume the whole fruit and vegetable and not simply take vitamin supplements.

Foods rich in antioxidants include almost all fruits and vegetables; they contain beta-carotene (converted to vitamin A in the body), vitamin C, and vitamin E. Regular intake of fruits and vegetables appreciably lowers your risk of developing cancer.[5] The National Research Council currently recommends the consumption of five servings of fresh fruit and vegetables

[4]L. Holmberg, E. M. Ohlander, and T. Byers. Diet and breast cancer risk. Results from a population-based, case-control study in Sweden. *Archives of Internal Medicine* 154: 1805–11, 1994.

[5]J. H. Weisburger. Nutritional approach to cancer prevention with emphasis on vitamins, antioxidants, and carotinoids. *American Journal of Clinical Nutrition* 53: 226S–37S, 1991.

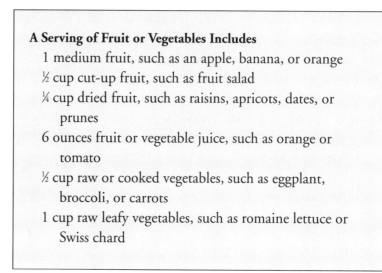

A Serving of Fruit or Vegetables Includes

1 medium fruit, such as an apple, banana, or orange

½ cup cut-up fruit, such as fruit salad

¼ cup dried fruit, such as raisins, apricots, dates, or prunes

6 ounces fruit or vegetable juice, such as orange or tomato

½ cup raw or cooked vegetables, such as eggplant, broccoli, or carrots

1 cup raw leafy vegetables, such as romaine lettuce or Swiss chard

daily. Unfortunately, only 10 percent of the U.S. population actually consumes that amount. Fruits and vegetables offer many similar nutrients, but vegetables contain a wider assortment of vitamins and minerals than do fruits.

Beta-carotene. Among the 600 or more carotenoids in foods, beta-carotene, lycopene, and lutein are the leaders in reducing the damage from free radicals. Foods high in beta-carotene are generally yellow or orange in color: cantaloupe, carrots, sweet potatoes, and winter squash. Lycopene, found in high quantities in tomatoes, is one of the most powerful antioxidants. Broccoli is also a rich source of beta-carotene. It appears to protect against many cancers, including cancer of the mouth, pharynx, esophagus, stomach, colon, rectum, prostate, and cervix. Lutein is found in broccoli, Brussels sprouts, grapefruit, kale, spinach, and watermelon.

Vitamin E. Vitamin E protects the body from cell damage that can lead to cancer, heart disease, and cataracts. Vitamin E works together with other antioxidants, such as vitamin C, in protecting from many chronic diseases. Vitamin E is found in vegetable oils, wheat germ, whole-grain products, seeds, nuts, and peanut butter. If you are trying to maintain a very low-fat diet, you should be cautious about increasing some of these foods. Speak to your health-care provider to see if a vitamin E supplement may be appropriate for you.

Vitamin C. The most famous antioxidant is vitamin C, and its touted benefits are well known. Current research has shown that vitamin C helps lower blood pressure and cholesterol, and it prevents many cancers, strokes, heart attacks, and diabetes. Foods rich in vitamin C are fruits (especially citrus fruits such as oranges and grapefruit), sweet peppers, broccoli, and potatoes.

FOOD SOURCES OF ANTIOXIDANTS

Beta-carotene	*Vitamin E*	*Vitamin C*
Acorn squash	Nuts	Broccoli
Broccoli	Peanut butter	Cantaloupe
Butternut squash	Seeds	Grapefruit
Brussels sprouts	Vegetable oils	Kiwi
Cantaloupe	Wheat germ	Oranges
Carrots	Whole-grain breads	Potatoes
Grapefruit	Whole-grain cereals	Strawberries
Kale		Sweet peppers
Spaghetti squash		Tangerines
Spinach		
Sweet potatoes		
Tomatoes		
Watermelon		

Alcohol and Breast Cancer Some evidence suggests that alcohol consumption increases the risk of developing breast cancer.[6] This effect appears to be linear, which means the more alcohol you consume, the higher your risk. Women with a high risk of developing breast cancer should consider abstain-

---

[6]S. A. Smith-Warner, D. Spiegelman, S. S. Yaun, et al. Alcohol and breast cancer in women: A pooled analysis of cohort studies. *Journal of the American Medical Association* 279: 535–40, 1998.

ing from alcohol, since an intake of just a few drinks per week can increase that risk. In general, the incidence of all cancers begins to rise with intake of as few as 2 drinks per day, so it is best to drink alcohol only in moderation.

Hormone Replacement Therapy and Cancer Risk Evidence also suggests that postmenopausal estrogen use increases the risk of breast cancer. The Nurses' Health Study (1976–92), representing 16 years of follow-up of nurses taking hormone replacement therapy, is one of the best studies to date.[7] During that time period 69,000 postmenopausal women were followed long-term and their risk of developing breast cancer along with their use of hormones was evaluated. It was found that women who used hormones long-term—10 or more years—were one and a half times as likely to develop breast cancer as those who did not take hormones. By virtue of the large numbers of women studied and the careful analysis by the investigators, the study has great credibility, and the increased risk of breast cancer found by it is quite significant. However, other smaller studies have failed to fully confirm these findings.

You should realize that taking hormone replacement therapy is beneficial to your health because of its prevention of heart disease and osteoporosis even though a relationship exists between estrogen use and breast cancer. Therefore, you need to make a decision about what is right for you as an individual. Some women should consider hormone replacement therapy, especially if they have strong family or personal risk factors for cardiovascular disease or osteoporosis. For example, if heart disease has caused early deaths in a family, hormone therapy may be warranted. However, if a mother and sister have been diagnosed with breast cancer at some point in their lives, the risk may be too high. I continue to advise hormone

[7]G. A. Colditz, S. E. Hankinson, D. J. Hunter, et al. Use of estrogens and progestins and the risk of breast cancer in postmenopausal women. *New England Journal of Medicine* 332: 1589–93, 1995.

replacement therapy for certain women, as long as they fully understand the risks and benefits. No one correct or easy answer to the hormone replacement therapy question exists.

Phytoestrogens and Breast Cancer Phytoestrogens are naturally occurring chemicals that are derived from plants and form part of our diet. They have a structure similar to estrogen, so the worry arises: Do these natural estrogens increase the risk of breast cancer? Luckily, phytoestrogens have an anticarcinogenic activity. A recent study actually found a substantial reduction in breast cancer in women ingesting phytoestrogens, and the more they ingested, the greater the protective effect.[8] So consuming soy is a simple and easy way to prevent breast cancer. Many of the recipes in this book are based on soy and will give you some good ideas on healthful, simple, and delicious ways to eat tofu and miso.

[8]D. Ingram, K. Sanders, and M. Kolybaba. Case-control study of phytoestrogens and breast cancer. *Lancet* 350: 990–94, 1997.

Chapter 8

Snacks, Foods on the Go, and Eating Out

Y ou may not always have time to cook complete meals now that you are menopausal, just as you may not have had time throughout your life. Many postmenopausal women are working, raising children, and busy with life's many commitments. Eating healthful foods on the go is important, since cooking full meals is not always possible. In addition, eating out is a pleasure that should not make you feel guilty. By following a few simple guidelines, you can eat out often and enjoy it. This chapter provides some tips and ideas for snacks, healthful foods on the go, and eating out.

Snacks

If you are so busy that you miss a meal or become hungry between meals, snacks can provide some good nutrition and an energy booster if you choose wisely. Avoid candy bars for snacks. If you are forced to eat from a vending machine, you can often select heart-healthy choices, which are labeled. At times like this, pretzels or popcorn and a seltzer or diet soda are a good choice. Planning ahead with snacks can really be a help. In that way you might even get in a quick phytoestrogen boost, with such snacks as roasted soynuts. And a piece of fruit is always fine.

The following table contains some ideas for snacks.

SNACKS

Fresh fruit	Dried fruit	Seeds, nuts and grains	Breads	Cookies	Dairy products
Apples	Apples	Almonds	Bagels	Fig bars	Cottage cheese
Bananas	Apricots	Low-fat granola	Graham crackers	Hermits	Frozen yogurt
Grapefruit	Banana chips	Dried fruit and nut mix	Low-fat crackers	Low-fat cookies	Low-fat ice cream
Grapes	Dates	Popcorn	Matzo		Soy yogurt
Melon	Figs	Pretzels	Melba toast		Yogurt
Nectarines	Pineapple	Pumpkin seeds	Whole-grain bread		
Oranges	Prunes	Soy nuts			
Peaches	Raisins	Sunflower seeds			
Pears		Walnuts			
Pineapple					
Plums					

Foods on the Go

The meals that you eat while you are away from home or that you bring to work do not need to be elaborate to be nutritious. Many of the meals in this book make superb lunches when reheated in the microwave. Leftovers from the previous night's dinner can make a simple and nutritious lunch. Invest in some microwave-safe plastic containers with lids and set aside the leftovers in these containers to take with you to work or while you are away from home the next day. Use some of the soy-based salad dressings (see Recipes, pages 91-303) and pack a crisp salad. Be sure to refrigerate these meals adequately to prevent bacterial contamination.

With a little planning, you can stock your refrigerator and cupboard with the components you need to pack meals on the go. See the Shopping List below of ingredients for nutritious dishes you can eat if you do not have time to cook or if you would like to pack a brown-bag meal to carry with you. All breads may be kept in the freezer. Buy less ripe fruit if you do not plan to use it immediately. Plan ahead when you shop.

SHOPPING LIST

Breads and grains	Protein sources	Fruits & vegetables	Extras	Phytoestrogen-rich foods
Bagels	Canned salmon	Soybean sprouts	Balsamic vinegar	Soy dogs
English muffins	Canned tuna	Avocados	Honey	Soy bread
Low-fat crackers	Cheese wedges	Baking potatoes	Jams	Soy drinks
Pita	Eggs	Bananas	Mustard	Soy burgers
Pretzels	Low-fat cottage cheese	Cucumbers	Olive oil	Soy cheddar cheese
Whole-grain bread	Low-fat cream cheese	Seasonal fruit	Red-wine vinegar	Soy cream cheese
	Sliced turkey	Romaine lettuce		Soy jack cheese
		Tomatoes		Soy mayonnaise
				Soy milk (plain, chocolate, strawberry)
				Soy pasta
				Soy yogurt
				Soy-nut butter

The following combination of the ingredients found in the Shopping List constitute healthful meals for postmenopausal women that fit in with their busy lifestyle.

Turkey and soy cheddar cheese on whole-grain bread with mustard, lettuce, and tomato; fresh fruit. The turkey provides a low-fat protein source, and substituting soy cheddar cheese for traditional cheese adds a phytoestrogen boost. Round it out with whole-grain bread for complex carbohydrates and fiber. Use mustard instead of mayonnaise to keep the fat content low. Have some fresh fruit for dessert to add some antioxidants.

Low-fat cheese (2 ounces), bagel, and grapes. Many low-fat varieties of cheese now are available, including Swiss, goat, and part-skim mozzarella. You may not be able to taste the difference between them and the higher-fat varieties.

Hummus on pita with lettuce, tomato, and sprouts. If you do not have time to make your own phytoestrogen-rich hummus (see recipe for Tofu Parsley Hummus, page 142), many excellent hummus products are available commercially, but they generally will not contain phytoestrogens. Hummus can be low in fat and rich in protein, carbohydrates, and fiber.

Cantaloupe filled with cottage cheese, pretzels. Cantaloupe is rich in beta-carotene, while calcium and protein are supplied by the cottage cheese. Choose a low-fat cottage cheese and accompany this with pretzels for some carbohydrates. It's delicious and convenient.

Grilled soy cheese sandwich, popcorn. Soy cheddar tastes delicious and makes a wonderful grilled cheese sandwich. Accompany it with some popcorn and a refreshing soy drink.

Lean roast beef with soy cheddar, lettuce, and tomato on whole-grain bread; fresh fruit. If you choose lean roast beef and use mustard instead of mayonnaise, you can keep the fat content of this sandwich relatively low. Serve it with soy cheddar for a dose of phytoestrogens and on whole-grain bread for some fiber.

Low-fat cream cheese (Neufchatel), tomato, and cucumber sandwich. Low-fat cream cheese is convenient to have on hand

and a good source of protein. Make this sandwich on whole-grain bread to boost the fiber content.

Soy cream cheese with raisins, walnuts, and honey on a bagel. Soy cream cheese is a delicious and phytoestrogen-rich alternative to traditional cream cheese. Add some raisins, walnuts, and honey for a wonderful sweetness and spread it on bagels.

Soy jack cheese, avocado, tomatoes, and romaine lettuce on pita. Cheese and avocado have an affinity for one another, so why not substitute soy cheese to add a phytoestrogen punch? The tomatoes add some beta-carotene, while the romaine adds a bit of calcium.

Soy-nut butter and jelly sandwich on sliced whole-grain bread. A phytoestrogen-rich alternative to traditional peanut butter and jelly that is as simple and quick to prepare as it gets. Have it with a glass of soy milk (try chocolate, strawberry, and other flavors) for a double phytoestrogen punch.

Some soy products such as vegetarian or soy burgers are made with "soy-protein concentrate," which contains almost no isoflavones. These soy products do not have the phytoestrogen benefits of unprocessed soy products, such as tofu and miso. However, if you see "soy-protein isolate" on the label, the isoflavones are largely retained. So check the label carefully if you are eating some of the more "ready-made" soy products.

Eating Out

Eating out in restaurants should be a relaxing and social affair. With a bit of education and effort on your part, you also can eat a perfectly healthful diet for menopause and post-menopause. Eating out in restaurants requires a strategy in order to choose what's good for you on the menu. Using some basic guidelines, you can continue to eat out and enjoy doing so after menopause and still stick to the principals of healthful eating. You even can add some phytoestrogens to your diet in many restaurants.

Strategies to Use When Eating Out

❖

- Choose meals based upon vegetables, tofu, beans, seafood, poultry, and lean meat.
- Avoid meals based upon bacon, ham, or ribs.
- Look for meals that are grilled, seared, broiled, baked, barbecued, steamed, roasted, or poached.
- Avoid meals that are fried or contain unhealthful buzz-words, such as crispy, creamed, pan-fried, buttery, au gratin, escalloped, or hollandaise.
- Ask for your meal to be prepared light, with a minimal amount of added butter or oil.
- Always ask for salad dressing and butter on the side, so that you can determine how much goes on your salad, bread, or potato.
- If portions are large, share an entrée or ask for a doggie bag to avoid overeating.
- If ordering dessert, try fresh fruit or sorbet. Or consider ordering only one rich dessert for the whole table, with everyone trying a few bites.

Chinese Chinese food is an excellent choice because you will have no problem finding plenty of sources of phytoestrogens. The Chinese have been using tofu (also called bean curd) mixed with other meats or vegetables long before Westerners ever realized the benefits of that type of eating. Try tofu in the many creative combinations offered. Try the many delicious, clear-broth soups in which you will often find tofu. Dishes based upon lo mein or noodles are good choices. Enjoy plenty of white rice with other entrées. Choose vegetarian items as much as possible; you never can be sure how much of the meat is really fat. Avoid deep-fried and pan-fried dishes and stay away from egg rolls, spare ribs, chicken wings, and pot stickers. You should routinely order your food cooked light even if they tell you it is made with 100 percent vegetable oil.

Thai Thai food is another menopausal feast that you should eat often. It is very light and chock full of phytoestrogens. Pad thai is a traditional favorite—order the vegetarian version and you will be sure to get your day's dose of phytoestrogens from the tofu. Thai noodle soups are usually a very light, clear broth and often contain tofu along with another meat, fish, or vegetable. So feel free to indulge. Stay away from the deep-fried spring rolls, but you may find some steamed versions, such as fresh rolls, just as satisfying. Experiment with the many interesting stir-fried entrées, trying tofu in new and varied combinations. Enjoy plenty of white rice with all your meals. Avoid meals cooked with high-fat coconut milk.

Japanese Japanese noodle soups are an excellent choice; they are usually light and filled with fresh vegetables. They often contain phytoestrogens in the form of miso. Miso and tofu also are found in many stir-fries. Sushi is a healthy choice—choose fish rich in omega-three fatty acids, such as tuna, salmon, and mackerel. The vegetarian types of sushi are great for those who don't want to eat raw fish. The seaweed wrappings (nori) are a rich source of calcium. Stay away from tempura, which is fried.

Vegetarian You will generally have no problem finding phytoestrogen-rich meals in vegetarian restaurants. But be wary, since you cannot assume that all vegetarian cooking is low in fat. Be cautious of meals based upon cheese or nuts since those ingredients are very high in fat. Stick to selections in which the main ingredients are tofu, tempeh, miso, beans, and grains. Avoid fried foods, which can be common in vegetarian restaurants.

Italian You will not find many phytoestrogen-rich dishes in an Italian restaurant, but if you exert a little discretion Italian food can still be a good choice. Try to choose meals based upon vegetables and pasta. Be cautious of risotto, as it often contains butter. Order meat, chicken, and fish that is roasted, baked, or broiled, not fried. Beware of dishes that contain large amounts of cheese. Choose the traditional "red sauce" over a "white sauce," which may be much higher in fat. Beware of eggplant Parmesan, since it is often deep fried. Enjoy a large salad, adding a small amount of olive oil and vinegar but beware of eating too many olives, since they are high in fat.

Mexican Mexican food does not necessarily deserve the bad reputation it has received. If you order carefully, you can eat well in Mexican restaurants. Avoid refried beans (which are cooked in lard), cheese, and sour-cream garnishes. Burritos are a good choice, but stick to vegetarian or grilled-chicken fillings. You occasionally can find some tofu options for fillings, which adds some phytoestrogens. The carnitas (pork butt) or beef fillings are often high in fat. Fajitas are an excellent choice, especially those made with vegetables, seafood, or chicken. Watch out for tortilla chips, fried taco shells, or fried tostada shells—all are loaded with fat. Use guacamole in moderation, as it is often prepared with sour cream.

Pizza You probably will not find phytoestrogen-rich ingredients in a pizza, but it still can be a staple in your diet. Pizza is widely available and inexpensive. However, you will need to watch out for the fat-laden toppings: sausage, pepperoni, bacon, hamburger. Your safest bet is to stick to vegetarian or light-cheese toppings when it comes to ordering pizza. And always remember moderation—have one or two slices with a nice light salad, and your meal will be satisfying and complete.

Indian You probably will not find many phytoestrogen-rich options on an Indian menu, but Indian food tends to be low in saturated fat and cholesterol. Many of the dishes use a yogurt-based curry. Tandoori chicken or fish dishes are a good choice, since they are roasted in a clay oven and get their flavor from spices rather than oil. Vegetables and legumes are an important part of Indian cooking. Be wary of some bean dishes, though, since they may be high in hidden fat. Avoid korma dishes, which contain cream and nuts.

Middle Eastern You will not find many phytoestrogen-rich ingredients in Middle Eastern cuisine but often it is based on healthful beans and grains. Hummus and falafel are prepared from ground chickpeas, which are an excellent low-fat source of protein. Falafel, however, is deep-fried and best avoided. The sauces for these dishes are usually yogurt-based, which is fine. Hummus can contain a large amount of tahini (sesame-seed paste), which can add considerable fat to the dish, although it is high in calcium. Couscous and bulgur are excellent high-carbohydrate accompaniments to many Middle Eastern dishes. If you would like to eat meat, kebabs are a good choice since they are grilled and much of the fat drips into the fire.

Steak House Your days of eating steak for dinner are not over. Moderation is the key. Try to keep your consumption of steak at one meal to 4 ounces, the approximate size of a deck of cards. You will generally be served far more than that. Ask for a doggie bag. Trim all the fat. Ask for your baked potato with the butter on the side and then use only a minimal amount or none at all. Avoid french fries. Watch out for the salad dressings at the salad bar—they may have more fat than your entire meal contains.

Deli Sandwiches from a deli can be delicious and healthful, but you must follow a few basic rules. Lean turkey and roast beef are good choices but avoid corned beef and pastrami since they are loaded with fat, salt, and additives. For condiments choose mustard instead of mayonnaise. Rotisserie chicken is fine, especially if you remove the skin. Avoid egg salad, tuna salad, chicken salad, potato salad, macaroni salad, and coleslaw; they all are prepared with mayonnaise, which adds a very high amount of fat. Beware of marinated salads, such as bean salad and pasta salad, that contain oil-based dressings. Instead, opt for grilled vegetables, fruit salads, and fresh fruit for side dishes. Choose baked chips, pretzels, or popcorn.

Fast Food Be very wary when eating in fast-food chains. The meals are often filled with fat and cholesterol. If you want a hamburger, choose one that is flame-broiled and eat it without mayonnaise, sauce, or cheese (ketchup or mustard is fine). Grilled chicken is generally a better choice, but, again, stay away from toppings. Baked potatoes with a small amount of olive oil or butter that you add yourself are fine, but potatoes already prepared with cheese, bacon, or sour cream are poor choices. In general, choose items from the "light" menu. Avoid french fries, onion rings, and fish fillets.

Part 2

✦

Recipes

Introduction

At first glance it may seem a daunting task to incorporate soy foods and flaxseed into your daily diet. You may be familiar with some of the soy foods in the markets, such as tofu and tempeh, but unfamiliar with miso and phytoestrogen-rich flaxseed. You also may believe that since you now will be eating soy and flaxseed on a regular basis, you are going to have to prepare separate meals for your family and friends.

But think again. Our aim is to show that with an understanding of how best to use soy and flaxseed in cooking, and with a bit of creativity, incorporating them into your daily diet is no more challenging and takes no more time than your everyday cooking. Best of all, when you cook the delectable foods found in this book, such as Chicken with Cilantro and Scallions (page 244), Pan-Seared Salmon with Creamed Spinach and Lemon (page 261), Romaine Salad with Garlicky Beef and Creamy Avocado Dressing (page 171), and Cranberry-Orange Cloud Cookies (page 293), and begin creating your own delicious meals, you will find that soy and flaxseed are truly world-class foods and that your family and friends will love your cooking.

Cooking with Soy and Flaxseed

When we first began developing recipes with soy and flaxseed in them, we were unfamiliar with not only the products but also the best way to use them in the kitchen. Our first attempts were flavorless and unappetizing disasters. We thought the only method to prepare firm tofu was to pair it with Asian seasonings and stir-fry it in a wok. We never even had heard of silken tofu, let alone its unique ability to transform a bland sauce into a palate-pleasing delight. Our experiments with flaxseed were no more successful. When we finally ventured into tossing a few tablespoons into batters, our brownies were gooey and our breads too dense. Through trial and error, though, we were able to refine the proportions and cooking times of flaxseed-laced recipes and make delectable cookies, bars, and pizza doughs. By reading about the ways other cooks use them and through experimenting on our own, we began to create wonderful recipes and discovered how soy and flaxseed are best used in cooking.

Here is a list of the primary phytoestrogen-rich foods used in this book:

Tofu	Soy nuts
Silken tofu	Soy cheese
Tempeh	Miso
Whole soybeans	Shoyu
Soy milk	Flaxseed

Some of these foods may be familiar to you, while others may seem confusing. We discuss each one below, so you will recognize it in the store and have recipe ideas for it. Remember: It's not necessary to use all of these foods in a single recipe to reap the nutritional benefits soy and flaxseed provide and cook great-tasting food. Our approach not only makes cooking with them practical but also offers room to be creative by combining them with more familiar foods to vary the flavors and textures of a dish. It should be mentioned that this list includes only the foods that we believe combine the best of nutrition, flavor, and cooking qualities. It seems that every conventional product now has a soy equivalent. Many stores now carry soy dogs and burgers, soy sausage, soy cheeses and mayonnaises, and soy-based sour creams and yogurts. We have used soy sausage and cheeses in recipes and they work well. However, we are not big fans of some of the other soy products. Soy mayonnaise has a sour taste, and we prefer to make our own soy burgers. With new soy foods being developed regularly, it probably is best to keep an open mind and try those that sound appealing. With that said, let's take a closer look at the phytoestrogen-powerhouse foods found in this book and discuss how they can be incorporated into your cooking.

Tofu Tofu or bean curd comes from soy milk. It is made by adding nigari (a compound from sea water), calcium sulfate, and vinegar to soy milk. The excess moisture is removed, and the remaining curds are pressed into blocks. A 6-ounce serving of tofu provides 12 grams of protein, as well as 5 grams of fat and approximately 720 milligrams of calcium.

Tofu is bland-tasting and requires creativity and bold flavors to make it something special. Tofu acts like a sponge in absorbing flavors during cooking. It turns out especially well when paired with full-flavored seasonings, such as herbs, spices, vinegars, garlic, and onions. Tofu can be grilled, stewed, baked, stir-fried, and mashed. Firm and extra-firm tofu work well as a meat replacement in stir-fries, stews, sandwiches, and egg dishes. Soft tofu works well in spreads, desserts, and dressings.

Tofu is sold in the refrigerated section of most markets, packed in water in 1-pound blocks. Unopened tofu has a shelf life of about 3 months, but once the container is opened, it tends to spoil quickly. Store unused portions of tofu in your refrigerator, floating them in water. If you change the water daily, the tofu should last 1 week. Chinese markets often sell it in bulk containers. We do not recommend purchasing tofu in that manner, since it may not be as fresh and those containers may harbor harmful bacteria.

Silken Tofu Japanese-style silken tofu is the tofu that provides the cook with the most opportunities to be creative. When we began experimenting with silken tofu, we discovered the countless ways it can be used in recipes. We came up with many new ideas and experienced a "tofu awakening." Once you begin creating recipes with silken tofu, you will be amazed by its ability to transform dishes that we all once considered off-limits, such as creamy pasta sauces and rich salad dressings, into everyday fare. Silken tofu is the tofu to use when you are "hiding" tofu in recipes. When it is pureed in a blender or a food processor, it can be used in place of cream in soups and sauces. It makes creamy dressings, luscious puddings, and dense cheesecakes. It adds a wonderful consistency to dips and spreads and makes surprisingly rich mashed potatoes. Silken tofu is available in firm and soft varieties packed in 12.3-ounce aseptically sealed containers in the refrigerated section of most markets.

Tempeh Tempeh is made from whole soy beans that first are cooked and then fermented and pressed into a dry and dense cake. Tempeh has a nutty flavor and chewy texture. Ounce for ounce, tempeh contains about twice the amount of calories and protein in tofu. A 7-ounce portion of tempeh has 395 calories, 38 grams of protein, 34 grams of carbohydrates, and 15 grams of fat.

In the kitchen tempeh works best in stir-fries, sandwiches, braised dishes, and on the grill. Its firm texture holds up well to stirring and long cooking, and, like tofu, it absorbs flavors well. Tempeh is available in vacuum-packed 8-ounce blocks in the refrigerated section of most markets. Once opened, tempeh should be used within 2 to 3 days.

Whole Soybeans Whole soybeans are mature beans that have been picked and dried. They are yellowish and similar in size to navy beans. The nutritional profile of soybeans is significantly different from that of other dried beans. Soybeans contain approximately twice as much protein as other beans and half the amount of carbohydrates. Also, 1/2 cup of cooked soybeans has approximately 5 grams of unsaturated fat, significantly more than the 1/2 gram that the average bean contains. Dried soybeans are not as readily available as other beans. Many natural foods stores stock them, and some large markets carry them in 1-pound packages. Canned soybeans are widely available in 14-ounce containers and are an excellent alternative.

Dried soybeans are prepared like other dried beans. They first need to be sorted, rinsed, and soaked for 8 hours. Their soaking water is then drained and discarded. They then are covered with fresh water and simmered for 3 hours. Even after such a long cooking time, they will retain a firm texture. Their texture is similar to chickpeas. They will never cook to the tenderness of pinto beans and kidney beans. Once cooked, soybeans can be added to soups and stews or pureed to make estrogen-rich spreads.

Soy Milk This liquid from cooked and pureed soybeans contains no cholesterol, is a fair source of calcium (many are calcium fortified), and is high in protein and plant estrogens. It is available in whole, low-fat, and nonfat varieties as well as sweetened and unsweetened. Some markets carry chocolate- and strawberry-flavored soy milk. You can purchase fresh soy milk in the dairy section of many markets or on the dry good shelves in airtight containers. Fresh soy milk will last a week in your refrigerator; the airtight containers about 3 months in your pantry.

The easiest way to incorporate soy milk in your diet is to

drink it, but its bland and nutty flavor is not for everyone. We like to substitute unsweetened soy milk in recipes for cow's milk. For example, to prepare wonderful, soy milk–based garlic mashed potatoes, simmer garlic in soy milk and puree the mixture with silken tofu. This base, when mashed with yellow-flesh potatoes makes a great dish. Soy milk also can be used in drinks, sauces, soups, and desserts.

Soy Nuts When whole soybeans are soaked in water and then dry roasted, the resulting product is known as soy nuts. They resemble peanuts, and like peanuts, they are high in protein and, unfortunately, high in fat as well. They are available in 1-pound packages in health food stores, and occasionally they are sold in bulk in larger markets. Although they do not spoil quickly, we still suggest buying only the amount you will immediately use.

Soy nuts are turned into a spicy snack when they are toasted in the oven with a dash of cayenne and a drizzling of chili oil. You also can grind them and add them to cookies or energy bars or try substituting them for peanuts or cashews in Asian-inspired dishes. Sprinkle them on just before serving so they maintain their crunch.

Soy Cheese Soy cheese is made from soy milk. It is a wonderful source of protein, calcium, and phytoestrogens. It is similar to dairy cheese in texture and usage but it is lower in fat. Some of the varieties include: mozzarella, jack, cheddar, cream cheese, and Parmesan. Mozzarella, jack, and cheddar are available in 12-ounce blocks. Cream cheese and Parmesan are sold in plastic containers.

Soy cheeses melt wonderfully and can be substituted for dairy cheese in recipes. All but soy Parmesan are used throughout this book. We continue to use traditional Parmesan, since small amounts generally are used, and we prefer the flavor.

Miso Japanese in origin and made from fermented soybeans, salt, and often rice or barley, miso has the consistency of soft butter and a rich and salty flavor. It is an excellent source of protein and B vitamins. However, it is high in sodium as well with approximately 900 milligrams in a tablespoon.

Miso is available in a variety of colors ranging from dark brown to yellow. Dark miso is virtually pure soybean and has an intense flavor. Lighter misos contain grains and are more mildly flavored. Since dark miso is pure soybean, it is a better source of plant estrogens than the lighter varieties. Miso is generally available in 8-ounce or 1-pound containers in health food stores or Asian markets.

Whisk miso into hot water, add a few cubes of tofu and a sprinkling of scallions and cilantro, and you have prepared an easy estrogen-rich meal. Miso also finds its way into salad dressings, marinades, and stews.

Shoyu Many commercially produced soy sauces are not fermented and are derived from hydrolyzed vegetable protein, corn syrup, caramel color, salt, and MSG. Shoyu, Japanese in origin, is a naturally fermented soy sauce containing only soybeans, wheat, and salt. It is the seasoning we prefer to use. If you cannot find it, tamari is a good substitute. Tamari is the Chinese version of shoyu and is sometimes made without wheat. Again, look in Asian markets and health food stores if you cannot find it in your supermarkets.

Flaxseed Although not a common food in America, flaxseed regularly is used in the kitchens in Scandinavia and Asia. Flaxseed can be considered a superfood. It is high in soluble fiber, protein, calcium, and potassium.

In this cookbook flaxseed most often is used as a baking ingredient. It is the main ingredient in Estro Bars (see page 298) and can be added to leavened doughs to produce wonderfully earthy breads and unique-tasting pizza doughs. When using flaxseed in baking, you will need little or no added fats, since flaxseed adds moisture to your baked goods. With flaxseed as a major ingredient, you will be able to make moist brownies, gingerbread, muffins, and cookies with virtually no oil or butter.

In a few instances you can use whole flaxseed, such as in a bread dough, but most often it is ground to resemble flour. The best tool for processing flaxseed is a coffee bean grinder. You can process a 1/2 cup of flaxseed in seconds to use in your recipes. Since ground flaxseed loses nutrients quickly, we suggest only grinding the flaxseed that you are going to use immediately.

Flaxseed is available in natural groceries and health food stores either in bulk containers or 1-pound packages. Like all seeds, flaxseed contains a significant amount of oil, and it can turn rancid quickly. Therefore, purchase flaxseed in small amounts (1–2 pounds) and keep it refrigerated.

Chapter 9

Drinks and Smoothies

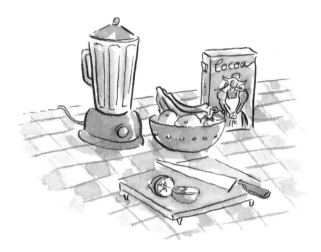

Consuming soy drinks is a quick and simple way to incorporate large amounts of phytoestrogens into your diet. We are not simply talking about drinking soy milk, but indulging in guilt-free smoothies and frappés. All of our drinks contain silken tofu, and many also feature soy milk and yogurt, which further boost your intake of phytoestrogens and calcium. Whether you choose to make one of our drinks for a breakfast on the go, a quick snack, or even a dessert, you will be amazed at how simple they are to prepare. With fruit, fruit juice, soy milk, tofu, and a blender or food processor you can create luscious drinks in just five minutes.

Cool off with the Citrus Delight, a refreshing blend of lemon sherbert, vanilla yogurt, and orange juice. You may think you are drinking a beverage prepared with premium ice cream, but it is silken tofu that provides the creamy taste and texture. Indulge in our Hot Cocoa, a rich combination of soy milk, cocoa, and silken tofu. If strawberries are a favorite fruit of yours, you may enjoy our Strawberry-Banana Smoothie, a no-fuss preparation of a banana, strawberries, and orange juice.

Allow our recipes to be your inspiration to create your own delicious drinks. By following a few guidelines, you will find preparing drinks to be an easy and rewarding experience. For smoothies, a banana adds a creamy texture and helps in binding the other ingredients. One or two ice cubes provide a frozen, slushy texture. The silken tofu makes it creamy. For frappés low-fat yogurt adds body, while extracts and syrups provide flavor, and silken tofu adds a creamy, rich texture. With just soy milk and a flavoring, warm drinks can be prepared in minutes. Some winning combinations are soy milk and almond extract, or soy milk, maple extract, and a touch of maple syrup. As you can see, creating your own phytoestrogen- and calcium-rich soy drinks is a breeze.

Strawberry–Banana Smoothie

Preparation: 5 minutes
Yield: 2 8-ounce
servings

Silken tofu adds creaminess as well as phytoestrogens to this cool and refreshing smoothie.

1 large banana
1 cup frozen strawberries
2 ice cubes
6 ounces silken tofu
½ cup orange juice

1. Place the banana, strawberries, ice, tofu, and orange juice in a blender or the work bowl of a food processor fitted with a metal blade.

2. Pulse the ingredients 5 times. Then process until a smooth drink forms.

3. Pour the smoothie into 2 glasses and serve immediately.

Peach–Berry Cooler

Silken tofu and yogurt make this frozen drink both phytoestrogen and calcium rich, a perfect way to cool your hot flashes.

Preparation: 5 minutes
Yield: 2 12-ounce
servings

1 cup frozen blueberries
1 cup frozen strawberries
1 large banana
1½ cups peach or apple juice
6 ounces silken tofu
4 ounces vanilla yogurt

1. Place the blueberries, strawberries, banana, peach or apple juice, tofu, and yogurt in the work bowl of a food processor fitted with a metal blade.

2. Pulse the ingredients 5 times. Then process until a smooth drink forms. Pour the drink into 2 glasses and serve immediately.

Citrus Delight

You can drink your hot flashes away with this sherbert cooler. Soy milk, silken tofu, and yogurt make it rich in phytoestrogens and calcium.

Preparation: 5 minutes
Yield: 2 8-ounce
servings

½ pint lemon sherbert
4 ounces nonfat vanilla yogurt
1 cup soy milk
6 ounces silken tofu
⅓ cup orange juice

1. Place the sherbert, yogurt, soy milk, tofu, and orange juice in the work bowl of a food processor fitted with a metal blade.

2. Pulse the ingredients 3 or 4 times. Then process until a smooth drink forms. Pour the drink into 2 glasses and serve immediately.

Chocolate Frappé

Preparation: 5 minutes
Yield: 2 8-ounce
servings

Chocolate frappés can be healthful and delicious! This one contains soy milk, chocolate frozen yogurt, and silken tofu, so you can cool your craving for chocolate without guilt. Tip: *The ingredients can be altered to create a variety of frappés. For a strawberry frappé, substitute strawberry frozen yogurt and strawberry yogurt; for a vanilla version, vanilla frozen yogurt and vanilla yogurt.*

½ **pint low-fat chocolate frozen yogurt**
6 ounces silken tofu
4 ounces low-fat chocolate yogurt
1 cup soy milk
2 tablespoons chocolate syrup

1. Place the frozen yogurt, tofu, yogurt, soy milk, and chocolate syrup in the work bowl of a food processor fitted with a metal blade.

2. Pulse the ingredients 3 or 4 times. Then process until a smooth frappé forms. Pour the frappé into 2 glasses and serve immediately.

Orange–Banana Creme

Preparation: 5 minutes
Yield: 2 12-ounce
servings

This refreshing thick shake is a healthful version of a banana Creamsicle. It contains yogurt, soy milk, and silken tofu, so it is rich in phytoestrogens and calcium yet low in fat.

½ pint orange sherbert
1 banana
4 ounces nonfat vanilla yogurt
1 cup soy milk
6 ounces silken tofu
1/3 cup orange juice

1. Place the sherbert, banana, yogurt, soy milk, tofu, and orange juice in the work bowl of a food processor fitted with a metal blade.

2. Pulse the ingredients 3 or 4 times. Then process until a smooth drink forms. Pour the drink into 2 glasses and serve immediately.

The Southern Peach

This refreshing peach cooler is thickened with silken tofu for a phytoestrogen boost. It is cool, creamy, and refreshing, and no one will know that it contains tofu unless you tell them!

Preparation: 5 minutes
Yield: 2 12-ounce servings

2 cups frozen peaches, peeled
1 large banana
1½ cups peach juice
6 ounces silken tofu

1. Place the peaches, banana, peach juice, and tofu in the work bowl of a food processor fitted with a metal blade.

2. Pulse the ingredients 5 times. Then process until a smooth drink forms. Pour the drink into 2 glasses and serve immediately.

The Hawaiian Pineapple

This pineapple cooler is so delicious that you never will make it any other way except with silken tofu. The banana balances the acidity of the pineapple and adds just the right amount of sweetness.

Preparation: 5 minutes
Yield: 2 12-ounce servings

2 cups frozen pineapple cubes
1 large banana
1½ cups pineapple juice
6 ounces silken tofu

1. Place the pineapple, banana, pineapple juice, and tofu in the work bowl of a food processor fitted with a metal blade.

2. Pulse the ingredients 5 times. Then process until a smooth drink forms. Pour the drink into 2 glasses and serve immediately.

Vanilla–Banana Creme

Preparation: 5 minutes
Yield: 2 12-ounce
servings

Creamy and intensely vanilla tasting, this drink is a great source of phytoestrogens and calcium.

½ pint low-fat vanilla frozen yogurt
1 banana
6 ounces silken tofu
4 ounces nonfat vanilla yogurt
1 teaspoon pure vanilla extract
1 cup soy milk

1. Place the frozen yogurt, banana, tofu, yogurt, vanilla extract, and soy milk in the work bowl of a food processor fitted with a metal blade.

2. Pulse the ingredients 3 or 4 times. Then process until a smooth frappé forms. Pour the frappé into 2 glasses and serve immediately.

Almond–Vanilla Blast

Intense flavors, such as almond and vanilla, work well with tofu. This slightly sweet and smooth-tasting drink is a great source of phytoestrogens and calcium.

Preparation: 5 minutes
Yield: 1 8-ounce
serving

1 large banana
¼ teaspoon almond extract
½ teaspoon vanilla extract
1–2 tablespoons maple syrup
8 ounces soy milk
2 ice cubes

1. Place the banana, almond extract, vanilla extract, maple syrup, soy milk, and ice cubes in the work bowl of a food processor fitted with a metal blade.

2. Pulse the ingredients 3 or 4 times. Then process until a smooth drink forms. Pour the drink into a glass and serve immediately.

Hot Cocoa

The next time you feel chilled, warm up with this rich and delicious drink. Prepared with soy milk and silken tofu, it is a phytoestrogen powerhouse. Tip: It may be necessary to stop processing the tofu after 30 seconds to scrape the tofu bits back toward the blade. Any bit of tofu that doesn't get pureed will float on the surface of the drink.

Preparation: 5 minutes
Cooking: 5 minutes
Yield: 2 8-ounce
servings

4 ounces silken tofu
12 ounces soy milk
2 tablespoons cocoa powder
2 tablespoons raw sugar
2 tablespoons brown-rice syrup

1. Place the tofu in a food processor fitted with a metal blade. Puree until it resembles whipped cream. Set aside.

2. Place the soy milk in a small sauce pan over low heat. Heat until it is very warm.

3. Whisk in the cocoa, sugar, and brown-rice syrup.

4. Whisk in the tofu and continue to heat the drink until it is very warm, but not boiling.

5. Divide the drink between 2 mugs.

Chapter 10

Breakfast

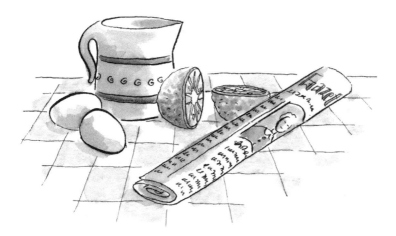

Since you were a child you have been told that breakfast is the most important meal of the day. Eating breakfast gives you the energy to face mental and physical challenges throughout the day. The obstacle is time—you never seem to have enough of it to prepare a healthful breakfast. In order to increase the amount of phytoestrogens at breakfast, it is necessary to be creative with your first meal of the day. Who wants to eat tofu or flaxseed for breakfast? We found that you can create tasty and phytoestrogen-powered breakfasts if you plan ahead. On the weekend prepare Estro Bars (see Sweets and Goodies chapter), a batch of Chocolate Cinnamon Granola, a loaf of New England Breakfast Bread, or even a recipe of Broccoli, Egg, and Cheddar Breakfast Roll-

Ups, which you can refrigerate and microwave for a minute or two on the following day. In this manner you can enjoy quick and delicious, phytoestrogen-rich breakfasts all week long.

Scrambled Eggs with Sausage, Scallions, and Tomatoes

Preparation: 10 minutes
Cooking: 10 minutes
Yield: 4 main-course servings

Eggs and sausage as part of a healthful menopause diet? Yes, eggs in moderation can be part of a heart-healthy diet. Since all of the cholesterol in an egg is in the yolk, our standard technique in eating eggs is always to use twice as many whites as eggs, which decreases the fat and cholesterol considerably. The addition of tofu to the eggs increases the yield of the recipe. In the end, only 2 egg yolks are in 4 servings! Both the sausage and cheese are soy-based, making this a triple-rich phytoestrogen meal. Try it on your family and friends and see if they notice the missing fat and cholesterol. Tips: *A nonstick skillet is the best pan for this recipe. Keep the heat high when you are cooking the eggs, and they will be done in approximately 4 minutes.*

2 eggs
4 egg whites
8 ounces firm tofu, mashed
Sea salt to taste
Black pepper to taste
1 tablespoon canola oil
6 ounces soy sausage, chopped
4 scallions, trimmed and sliced
1 tomato, cored and diced
2 ounces soy cheddar, sliced or grated

1. Whisk together the eggs, egg whites, and tofu. Season with sea salt and black pepper.

2. Heat the oil in a nonstick skillet over medium heat. Add the chopped sausage to the pan and cook until browned, stirring occasionally.

3. Reduce the heat to low and add the scallions to the pan. Cook until soft. Add the tomato to the pan and cook all the ingredients for 2 minutes.

4. Raise the heat to high. When the pan is hot, pour in the egg mixture. Allow the eggs to set for 30 seconds and then stir them often until firm. Stir in the soy cheddar and cook the eggs for 30 seconds more. Season with sea salt and black pepper.

5. Divide the eggs among 4 plates and accompany with toasted bagels.

Sea Salt

Salt is an often overlooked ingredient in cooking. A friend once said that knowing how to cook is knowing how to use salt and pepper. Just as freshly ground pepper is essential to good food, so is salt.

Sea salt is made from evaporated sea water. Common table salt has been highly processed, contains additives to keep it free-running, and only adds a salty flavor to your food. Sea salt is minimally processed and will draw out and intensify the flavors in your cooking. It is available in many natural food stores and through the mail from specialty food companies. Coarse-grained kosher salt is also an additive-free salt and is a good substitute.

Tomato and Egg

While this garlicky egg and tomato dish makes a fine breakfast, it also is a favorite Sunday evening supper of ours. We double the ratio of egg whites to egg yolks to keep the meal low in cholesterol and fat. As with the previous recipe, tofu is added to the eggs to provide a source of phytoestrogens. Tip: *When top-quality fresh*

Preparation: 15 minutes
Cooking: 5 minutes
Yield: 4 main-course servings

tomatoes are available, substitute them for the canned variety. They will need to be peeled and seeded.

    2 eggs
    4 egg whites
    8 ounces firm tofu, mashed
    Sea salt to taste
    Black pepper to taste
    1 tablespoon olive oil
    6 cloves garlic, peeled and sliced
    1 28-ounce can whole tomatoes, drained, seeded, and
      chopped
    4 bagels, halved

1. Whisk together the eggs, egg whites, and tofu and season with sea salt and black pepper.

2. Heat the olive oil in a nonstick skillet over low heat. Add the garlic to the oil and cook until soft and fragrant.

3. Raise the heat to high and add the tomatoes to the pan. Bring to a boil. Reduce the heat and simmer the tomatoes until all of their liquid has evaporated, stirring occasionally.

4. Raise the heat to high. When the pan is hot, pour in the egg mixture. Allow it to set for 30 seconds and then stir often until firm. Season with sea salt and black pepper.

5. Divide the eggs among 4 plates and accompany with the bagels.

Broccoli, Egg, and Cheddar
Breakfast Roll-Ups

Preparation: 15 minutes
Cooking: 10 minutes
Yield: 4 main-course
servings

These broccoli, egg, and cheese breakfast sandwiches use flour tortillas in place of the traditional English muffins for a welcome change. With broccoli, soy cheese, and tofu, the sandwiches are calcium and phytoestrogen rich.

Slicing Versus Mincing Fresh Garlic

From pasta and risotto to soup and stew, many memorable dishes begin with fresh garlic being cooked in olive oil. The aroma alone is enough to draw the curious toward the kitchen. However, it is not its smell but the incredible flavor that cooked garlic imparts to a dish that has given garlic its legendary status. What then is the best method to prepare garlic for cooking?

Until recently, we assumed that garlic needed to be minced to release the most flavor. However, we have found that although mincing does produce a strong garlic taste, often this flavor is bitter. Thinly slicing the garlic is a better choice. The garlic takes on a wonderfully sweet and intense flavor with no hint of bitterness or "bite."

1 cup water
Sea salt to taste
5 cups broccoli florets (reserve the stems for another use)
2 eggs
4 egg whites
8 ounces firm tofu, mashed
Black pepper to taste
1 tablespoon canola oil
3 cloves garlic, peeled and sliced
2 ounces soy cheddar, sliced or grated
4 large flour tortillas, warmed

1. Bring the water to a boil in a Dutch oven. Add a dash of sea salt. Place the broccoli flowers in the water, cover the pot, and steam the broccoli until it is tender, approximately 5 minutes. Drain and cool under running water.

2. Whisk together the eggs, egg whites, and tofu. Season with sea salt and black pepper.

3. Heat the oil in a nonstick skillet over medium heat. Add the garlic to the skillet. Cook the garlic until it is soft and fragrant. Add the broccoli. Cook the ingredients, stirring often, until the broccoli is hot.

4. Raise the heat to high. When the skillet is hot, pour in the egg mixture. Allow the eggs to set for 30 seconds and then stir often until firm. Stir in the soy cheddar and cook the eggs for 30 seconds more. Season with sea salt and black pepper.

5. Divide the eggs among the 4 tortillas. Roll the tortillas and serve at once.

Dutch Oven

One of the most versatile pots you can own is a Dutch oven. With its high sides and broad bottom, it is a cross between a stock pot and a sauté pan. In fact, it can be substituted for both. It can be used to cook pasta, make stock or soup, sear and braise meat or poultry, and prepare stir-fries. Dutch ovens come in a variety of materials, but an enameled cast-iron one is probably the best. With proper care, it will last a lifetime.

Blueberry–Filled French Toast Sandwiches

Preparation: 10 minutes
Cooking: 15 minutes
Yield: 4 main-course servings

In the past we prepared these breakfast French toast sandwiches with a cream cheese–based filling. Here we have substituted a tofu-based filling in order to add phytoestrogens and to lower the fat content. Although the consistency of a tofu-based filling is not as thick as the cream-based filling, the flavor is still wonderful.
Tips: *Experiment with different breads in this recipe. Sourdough, challah (which is higher in fat and calories), and honey wheat all*

work well. Also, if you use frozen blueberries, thaw and drain them before stirring them into the tofu.

6 ounces silken tofu

3 tablespoons maple syrup

3 tablespoons all-fruit blueberry jam

1 cup fresh or frozen (thawed and drained) blueberries

2 eggs

4 egg whites

1 cup soy milk

½ teaspoon cinnamon

8 ½-inch-thick slices crusty bread

4 teaspoons unsalted butter, divided

1. Combine the tofu, maple syrup, and jam in the work bowl of a food processor fitted with a metal blade. Process the ingredients until they are smooth. Transfer them to a bowl and stir in the fresh or frozen blueberries. Set the filling aside.

2. In a bowl whisk together the eggs, egg whites, soy milk, and cinnamon. Transfer to a shallow bowl.

3. Soak each slice of bread in the mixture until saturated. Melt 2 teaspoons of the butter in a large skillet over medium heat. When the butter sizzles, add 4 slices of bread. Cook the slices until they are lightly browned on each side and cooked through. Transfer to a warm plate. Repeat the procedure with the remaining butter and bread. Reduce the heat to low.

4. Spread a portion of the blueberry filling on 4 slices of the bread. Place the remaining slices over the filling to make sandwiches. Place the sandwiches in the pan and heat for 2 minutes, turning once.

5. With a serrated knife, cut each sandwich into 4 triangles. Divide the triangles among 4 plates. Accompany with warm maple syrup.

Soy Milk Pancakes

Preparation: 10 minutes
Cooking: 10 minutes
Yield: 2 main-course servings

Once you have tasted these distinctively flavored pancakes, you'll wonder why you haven't always made pancakes with soy milk. Soy milk pancakes are light and tender and taste better than their dairy counterparts. To make fruit pancakes, sprinkle the fruit on the pancakes once the bubbles have appeared. Tip: *If you use a well-seasoned cast-iron pan to cook your pancakes, you will need a minimal amount of butter.*

1 cup unbleached, all-purpose flour
2 teaspoons baking powder
½ teaspoon baking soda
½ teaspoon salt
1 tablespoon sugar
1 egg
1 cup soy milk
1 teaspoon vanilla extract
2 teaspoons canola oil
Unsalted butter for the pan
Maple syrup for drizzling

1. Heat the oven to 250°F. Heat a pan over medium-low heat.

2. In a large bowl whisk together the flour, baking powder, baking soda, salt, and sugar. Set the bowl aside.

3. In another bowl whisk together the egg, soy milk, vanilla extract, and canola oil.

4. Make a well in the center of the dry ingredients and pour the liquid ingredients into it. Whisk the batter until smooth.

5. Place a small amount of butter in the pan. Swirl it until it stops sizzling. Pour approximately 1/3 cup of batter into the pan. Cook the pancake until bubbles form on the surface, approximately 1 minute. Flip the pancake and cook it for another minute. Place it in the oven to keep it warm. Repeat the procedure with the remaining batter.

6. When all the pancakes have been cooked, divide them among 2 plates and accompany with maple syrup.

New England Breakfast Bread

Serve this hearty, nut-and-seed–laced bread for breakfast, spread with light cream cheese and fruit jam or thickly sliced for a sandwich. It is a good source of fiber and phytoestrogens. Tip: *This is a sticky dough. When kneading it, resist the temptation to add an excessive amount of flour.*

Preparation: 3½ hours
Cooking: 50 minutes
Yield: 1 loaf

THE SPONGE
1 tablespoon active dry yeast
¾ cup soy milk, warmed
1 cup unbleached white flour

REMAINING INGREDIENTS
⅓ cup plus 3 tablespoons flaxseed
1¼ cups warm (110°F) soy milk
½ cup whole-wheat flour
½ cup rolled oats
3 tablespoons poppy seeds
3 tablespoons sunflower seeds
1 cup raisins
4 tablespoons brown-rice syrup
1 teaspoon sea salt
3 cups unbleached white flour
Oil for the bowl and pan
1 egg white
1 teaspoon water

1. To prepare the sponge, combine the yeast and soy milk in a medium-sized bowl. Stir the ingredients until the yeast is dissolved and let the mixture rest for 10 minutes. Stir in the flour until the sponge is smooth. Let the sponge rest for 1 hour.

2. Grind ⅓ cup of flaxseed in a coffee grinder until it resembles flour. Set aside.

3. Add the whole-wheat flour, ground and whole flaxseeds, oats, poppy seeds, sunflower seeds, raisins, and brown-rice syrup to the sponge. Stir the ingredients until well incorporated.

4. Add the sea salt and ½ cup of the white flour and stir the ingredients well. Continue adding the flour ½ cup at a time, stirring until all of the flour is used.

5. Turn the dough out onto a lightly floured work surface. Knead for 15 minutes or until smooth and elastic. Add more flour to the work surface to keep the dough from sticking. This should be a sticky dough, so try not to add too much additional flour.

6. Place the dough in a very lightly oiled bowl. Turn the dough to coat the entire surface. Cover with plastic wrap and place in a warm and draft-free place until it is doubled in size, approximately 1½ hours.

7. Lightly oil a 9 x 5–inch loaf pan. Deflate the dough and turn it out onto a work surface. Form the dough into a loaf and place in the prepared pan. Cover with plastic wrap and allow to rise until it is doubled in size, approximately 1 hour.

8. Heat the oven to 350°F. Whisk together the egg white and water. Brush the loaf with the mixture. Bake the loaf for 50 minutes or until it reaches an internal temperature of 195°F. Remove the bread from the pan and allow it to cool on a wire rack.

Chocolate Cinnamon Granola

*Preparation: 15
minutes
Cooking: 10 minutes
Yield: 5 cups*

Traditional granola is high in fat. This low-fat version is also phytoestrogen rich, since it contains flaxseed. For a quick menopause breakfast, serve with soy milk and grab an Estro Bar on your way out. Tip: *When stirring the granola during its cooking, keep it in a single layer. If it is mounded, it won't toast well.*

1¾ cups regular oats (not quick cooking)

1 cup soy nuts

¾ cup flaxseed

2 tablespoons sesame seeds

4 tablespoons oat bran

2 teaspoons cinnamon

¼ teaspoon sea salt

1 cup barley malt

2 tablespoons maple syrup

⅔ cup chocolate chips

1. Heat the oven to 350°F. Heat a heavy skillet, preferably cast-iron, over medium-low heat. Add the oats and soy nuts and cook until the ingredients begin to toast, stirring occasionally, for approximately 5 minutes.

2. Add the flaxseed, sesame seeds, and oat bran and cook, stirring often for another 3 minutes. Add the cinnamon and sea salt to the skillet. Transfer to a heavy baking tray.

3. Combine the barley malt and maple syrup in a small saucepan. Gently bring the liquid to a boil.

4. Pour the liquid onto the granola and combine the ingredients thoroughly. Spread the granola in a single layer.

5. Bake the granola for 10 minutes, stirring every 3 minutes.

6. Remove the granola from the oven and transfer to a clean baking tray. Allow to cool for 5 minutes, then stir the chocolate chips into it. Cool for another 5 minutes, then crumble it with your fingers.

7. When the granola is cool, place it in an airtight container.

Cranberry–Pecan Granola

This hearty, flaxseed-based granola combines the tart flavor of cranberries with the sweetness of dried figs and raisins. It is wonderful to eat for breakfast by the handful or sprinkled on your favorite frozen yogurt.

Preparation: 15 minutes
Cooking: 10 minutes
Yield: 7 cups

2 cups regular oats (not quick cooking)
⅓ cup pecans, coarsely chopped
3 tablespoons sunflower seeds
¾ cup flaxseed
4 tablespoons oat bran
¼ teaspoon sea salt
1 cup brown-rice syrup
3 tablespoons barley malt
8 dried figs, sliced
¾ cup raisins
¾ cup dried cranberries

1. Heat the oven to 350°F. Heat a heavy skillet, preferably cast-iron, over medium-low heat. Add the oats, pecans, and sunflower seeds and cook until the ingredients begin to toast, stirring occasionally, for approximately 5 minutes.

2. Add the flaxseed and oat bran and cook, stirring often for another 3 minutes. Stir in the sea salt. Transfer the ingredients to a heavy baking tray.

3. Combine the brown-rice syrup and barley malt in a small saucepan. Gently bring the liquid to a boil.

4. Pour the liquid onto the granola and combine the ingredients thoroughly. Spread the granola in a single layer.

5. Bake the granola for 10 minutes, stirring every 3 minutes.

6. Remove the granola from the oven and transfer to a clean baking tray. Allow to cool for 5 minutes, then stir in the figs, raisins, and cranberries. Cool for another 5 minutes, then crumble it with your fingers.

7. When the granola is cool, place it in an airtight container.

Chapter 11

Soups

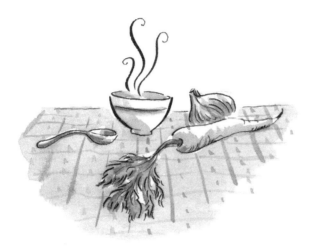

From a cook's perspective, nothing is more enjoyable than preparing homemade soups—except, of course, eating them. Delightful soups can be prepared with a minimal amount of ingredients. Some of the tastiest soups result from using your imagination and the odds and ends in your refrigerator. With an onion, garlic, a few root vegetables, a block of tofu, a tablespoon of miso, and a can of beans, you can make a wonderful soup. Although several of the soups in this chapter require an hour or two of cooking, the majority of that time the soup is simmering, needing little attention, just a stir now and then. You can go about your work and enjoy the wonderful aromas wafting from your kitchen.

Since we like to serve soups as a main course, ours are hearty and satisfying. We usually accompany them with a big green salad, crusty bread, and a small wedge of rich cheese. Like salad dressing and dips, soups are a great way to introduce soy into your diet. We like to use either cubed or pureed silken tofu in our soups. When it is cubed, it adds texture to broth-based soups. When it is pureed, it adds a delightful creaminess.

The soups in this chapter are prepared with a minimal amount of fat, offering balanced nutrition. Taking advantage of the winning combination of pureed potatoes and silken tofu, we have created Potato and Broccoli Soup and Kale, Collard, and Potato Soup. These rich-tasting soups are low in fat and incredibly high in phytoestrogens and calcium. In this chapter you will find broth-based soups, such as Tofu Meatball, Escarole, and Noodle Soup, and variations of traditional creamy favorites, such as Lentil Bisque. When you want a light and fast lunch, try the Quick Miso Soup—a fresh-tasting broth soup with cubed tofu, scallions, and cilantro.

We hope you will enjoy making these soups, allowing them to serve as an inspiration for creating your own estrogenic masterpieces.

Quick Miso Soup

Preparation: 5 minutes
Cooking: 10 minutes
Yield: 2 side-dish
servings

Miso is a fermented soy product that, like tofu, is a rich source of phytoestrogens. Bok choy is an excellent source of calcium. Tip: *This recipe can be multiplied. Also, 8 ounces of spinach is a wonderful addition to the soup. Add it 3 minutes after the bok choy.*

3 tablespoons dark miso
4 cups boiling water, divided
6 ounces bok choy, trimmed, stems sliced diagonally into
   ¾-inch thick pieces and leaves coarsely chopped
4 ounces silken tofu, cut into small cubes
½ teaspoon sugar

Sea salt to taste

Black pepper to taste

¼ cup cilantro, chopped

2 scallions, trimmed and thinly sliced

1. Place the miso on the bottom of a small Dutch oven. Whisk in ½ cup of the water. Whisk the miso and water together until the miso is dissolved.

2. Add the remaining water to the pot and bring the broth to a simmer. Add the bok choy and tofu to the broth and simmer for 5 minutes.

3. Add the sugar to the broth and season with sea salt and black pepper. Divide the broth among 2 bowls and garnish each serving with cilantro and scallions.

Potato and Broccoli Soup

This delicious and creamy soup gets its texture from tofu and soy milk, both excellent sources of phytoestrogens. In addition, the broccoli adds a healthful dose of calcium as well as antioxidants. Tips: Be sure to cook the broccoli enough to bring out its flavor, but not so much that it tastes like cabbage. Taste it immediately after it turns bright green and then once every minute until you are satisfied with the flavor. Also, the broccoli can be chopped either by hand or in a food processor fitted with a metal blade.

Preparation: 15 minutes
Cooking: 35 minutes
Yield: 4 main-course servings

1 tablespoon canola oil

3 cloves garlic, peeled and sliced

1 onion, peeled and diced

2–3 russet potatoes, scrubbed and cubed

Sea salt to taste

4 cups vegetable or chicken broth or water

1½ pounds broccoli, trimmed (cut off the bottom 2 inches of the stem and peel the remaining stem) and finely chopped

12 ounces silken tofu

1 cup soy milk

Black pepper to taste

1. Heat the oil in a Dutch oven over low heat. Add the garlic and cook until soft and fragrant. Add the onion and cook it until it is soft, stirring it occasionally.

2. Add the potatoes to the pot and sprinkle with sea salt. Cover the pot and steam the ingredients for 5 minutes, stirring occasionally.

3. Raise the heat to high and add the broth or water. Bring the liquid to a boil. Cover the pot, reduce the heat, and simmer the ingredients until the potatoes are tender, about 20 minutes.

4. Transfer the ingredients to the work bowl of a food processor fitted with a metal blade and puree the ingredients.

5. Return the puree to the pot over low heat and add the broccoli. Slowly heat the soup until the full broccoli flavor has developed, approximately 5 minutes, stirring often.

6. Combine the tofu and soy milk in the work bowl of the food processor and puree them. Stir the soy mixture into the soup. Season the soup with sea salt and black pepper. Ladle the soup into 4 bowls and accompany with rustic bread and a green salad.

Vegetable Broth

Preparation: 15 minutes
Cooking: 1³/₄ hour
Yield: 14 cups

This intensely flavored broth can be used as the base for many of the soups, stews, and sauces in this book. Also, with the addition of cubed silken tofu and chopped flat-leaf parsley or basil, it can be served as a first course or light lunch. The multitude of vegetables used in the broth's preparation enrich it with antioxidants, important in preventing many types of cancer. Tip: *Feel free to vary the vegetables in this recipe but avoid members of the cabbage family. They will overpower the broth.*

1 tablespoon canola oil
6 cloves garlic, peeled and sliced
1 leek, trimmed, washed, and sliced
2 scallions, trimmed and sliced

1 onion, peeled and chopped

8 ounces mushrooms, sliced

Sea salt to taste

1 gallon cold water, divided

2 carrots, peeled and chopped

2 parsnips, peeled and chopped

3 ribs celery (include some leaves), chopped

8 sprigs flat-leaf parsley

8 sprigs cilantro

1. Heat the oil in a stock pot over low heat. Add the garlic and cook until soft and fragrant, stirring often. Add the leek, scallions, onion, and mushrooms to the pot and sprinkle with sea salt. Raise the heat slightly and cook the vegetables for 5 minutes, stirring often.

2. Raise the heat to high and add 2 cups of water to the pot. Bring the water to a boil, reduce the heat, and simmer for 10 minutes.

3. Add the carrots, parsnips, celery, parsley, and cilantro to the pot. Add 2 more cups of water to the vegetables, bring the liquid to a boil, reduce the heat, and simmer for 10 more minutes.

4. Add the remaining water to the pot and bring the liquid to a boil. Reduce the heat and simmer the broth for 1 hour.

5. Allow the broth to cool slightly. Strain it into a large bowl and press the vegetables with the back of a spoon to extract as much liquid and flavor as possible. Refrigerate the broth until it is needed or freeze it in several small containers.

Kate's Lentil and Chickpea Soup with Root Vegetables and Couscous

The beans and root vegetables in this hearty soup are all rich sources of fiber, important in preventing colon cancer. Tempeh adds a wonderful texture and a good dose of phytoestrogens.

Although this soup requires 2 hours of cooking time, it doesn't

Preparation: 15 minutes
Cooking: 2 hours
Yield: 4 main-course
servings

need much attention, just a stir now and then. The long cooking time softens the vegetables and beans and allows their flavors to develop fully. Tip: *Stir this soup gently. Silken tofu has a tendency to lose its shape with vigorous stirring.*

1 tablespoon extra-virgin olive oil
4 cloves garlic, peeled and sliced
1 onion, peeled and diced
Sea salt to taste
2 ribs celery, diced
2 carrots, peeled and diced
1 parsnip, peeled and diced
1 potato, peeled and diced
1 small rutabaga, peeled and diced
½ cup green lentils, rinsed
1 15-ounce can chickpeas, drained and rinsed
8 cups water
8 ounces tempeh, cut into small cubes
⅔ cup Israeli couscous
8 ounces escarole, trimmed and chopped
Black pepper to taste

1. Heat the olive oil in a Dutch oven over medium heat. Add the garlic and cook until soft and fragrant, stirring often. Add the onion and sprinkle with sea salt. Cook the onion until soft, stirring often.

2. Reduce the heat to low and add the celery, carrots, parsnip, potato, rutabaga, lentils, and chickpeas to the pot. Stir the ingredients and cover the pot.

3. Steam the ingredients for 10 minutes. Raise the heat to high and add the water to the pot. Bring the soup to a boil and stir in the tempeh. Reduce the heat to a low simmer, cover the pot, and simmer the soup for 1½ hours.

4. Remove the pot from the heat and stir in the couscous and escarole. Season the soup with sea salt and pepper. Cover the pot and allow the soup to rest for 10 minutes.

5. Ladle the soup into 4 large bowls and accompany with crusty bread and, if desired, a green salad.

Israeli Couscous

Israeli couscous, like Moroccan couscous, is made from semolina. Israeli couscous is larger than the Moroccan variety, about the size of a peppercorn, and unlike the Moroccan type, it is toasted. Its large size and nutty flavor make it a versatile food. It can be cooked and tossed with vegetables and a vinaigrette to make a great chilled salad, or it can be added to soups and stews to absorb their wonderful juices. It also can be lightly seasoned and served as a bed for meat or fish.

Kale, Collard, and Potato Soup

Leafy greens, such as kale and collards, as well as the sea vegetable wakame are excellent sources of calcium. The tofu adds a creamy texture and phytoestrogens to this nutritious potato soup. Tip: We like to use vegetable broth in this soup. However, if you don't have any on hand, water or low-sodium canned chicken broth are fine substitutes.

Preparation: 15 minutes
Cooking: 35 minutes
Yield: 4 main-course servings

1 tablespoon olive oil
3 cloves garlic, peeled and sliced
1 onion, peeled and sliced
4 5-inch strips wakame
1 carrot, peeled and sliced
Sea salt to taste
½–⅔ pound green kale, trimmed, chopped, washed, and drained
½ pound collard greens, trimmed, washed, and drained
1 medium potato, scrubbed and diced
6–7 cups vegetable broth (see page 124) or water
Black pepper to taste
8 ounces silken tofu, pureed

1. Heat the olive oil in a Dutch oven over low heat. Add the garlic and cook until soft and fragrant. Add the onion and cook until soft.

2. Raise the heat slightly and add the wakame and carrot to the pot. Sprinkle the vegetables with sea salt. Cover the pot and steam the vegetables for 5 minutes, stirring occasionally.

3. Add the kale, collards, and potato to the pot. Cover the pot and steam the vegetables for 10 minutes, stirring occasionally.

4. Raise the heat to high and add the vegetable broth or water to the pot. Bring the soup to a boil. Reduce the heat, cover the pot, and simmer the soup until the potato is tender, approximately 20 minutes.

5. Carefully transfer the soup to the work bowl of a food processor fitted with a metal blade (it may be necessary to perform this procedure in 2 steps). Puree the soup.

6. Return the soup to the pot and season with sea salt and black pepper. Stir in the tofu.

7. Ladle the soup into 4 bowls and accompany with crusty bread and a small amount of rich cheese.

Split Pea Bisque

Preparation: 10 minutes
Cooking: 50 minutes
Yield: 4 main-course servings

This bisque is made creamy and uniquely flavored by the addition of the phytoestrogen-rich ingredients silken tofu and miso. Silken tofu is a low-fat and calcium-rich alternative to cream for thickening bisques. The split peas are a great source of fiber, important in the prevention of many cancers. Tip: *Prepare this soup a day in advance; gently reheat it the following day. As with many soups, this one is more flavorful on the second day.*

1 tablespoon canola oil
2 cloves of garlic, peeled and sliced
1 onion, peeled and diced
1 leek, washed, trimmed, and sliced
Sea salt to taste

1 carrot, peeled and diced

2 medium Yellow Finn or Yukon Gold potatoes, scrubbed
   and quartered

1½ cups split peas

2 tablespoons dark miso

7 cups water

6 ounces silken tofu, pureed

Black pepper to taste

1. Heat the oil in a Dutch oven over low heat. Add the garlic and cook until soft and fragrant. Add the onion and leek and sprinkle the ingredients with sea salt.

2. Cook the ingredients until the onion is soft. Add the carrot to the pot. Cover the pot and steam for 5 minutes.

3. Add the potatoes, split peas, and miso to the pot. Cook for 2 minutes.

4. Raise the heat to high and add the water to the pot. Bring the soup to a boil, cover the pot, and reduce the heat. Simmer until the split peas are tender, approximately 45 minutes.

5. Transfer the soup to the work bowl of a food processor fitted with a metal blade and puree the soup. Return it to the Dutch oven. Stir in the tofu. If necessary, add water to thin the soup to the desired consistency.

6. Season the soup with sea salt and black pepper. Ladle the soup into 4 bowls and accompany with crusty bread.

Lentil Bisque

Unlike a traditional bisque, which is finished with cream, our version uses silken tofu to provide a creamy flavor and texture. The result is a great-tasting and healthful soup that packs a phytoestrogen punch. In addition, the lentils are fiber-rich, important in preventing many cancers. Tips: *This soup is more flavorful on the second day. When reheating it, do so gently. High heat will curdle the soup. Also, this recipe calls for the garlic to be browned.*

Preparation: 15 minutes
Cooking: 50 minutes
Yield: 4 main-course servings

Since garlic cooked to the browning point has a tendency to burn quickly, monitor it closely.

4 tomatoes, cored and diced
1/3 cup flat-leaf parsley, chopped
1 tablespoon olive oil
8 cloves garlic, peeled and sliced
Sea salt to taste
1 onion, peeled and diced
1 bulb fennel, trimmed and diced
3 tablespoons dark miso
1½ cups green lentils, sorted and rinsed
6 cups water
8 ounces silken tofu
Black pepper to taste

1. Combine the tomatoes and parsley in a bowl and set them aside.

2. Heat the olive oil in a Dutch oven over medium heat. Add the garlic to the oil and sprinkle with sea salt. Cook the garlic until browned, approximately 4 minutes, stirring often.

3. Reduce the heat slightly and add the onion to the pot. Cook the onion until it is soft, stirring it occasionally. Add the fennel and miso and sprinkle with sea salt.

4. Cover the pot and steam the fennel until soft. Add the lentils to the pot and cook for 1 minute.

5. Raise the heat to high and add the water to the pot. Bring the soup to a boil. Reduce the heat and simmer the soup until the lentils are tender, approximately 40 minutes.

6. Place the tofu in the work bowl of a food processor fitted with a metal blade. Process the tofu until smooth and transfer to a bowl.

7. Transfer the soup to the food processor and puree it. Return the soup to the pot and stir in the tofu. Season with sea salt and black pepper.

8. Divide the soup among 4 bowls. Garnish each serving with the tomatoes and parsley. Accompany with crusty bread and, if desired, a small amount of rich cheese.

Tofu Meatball, Escarole, and Noodle Soup

This soup is based upon a recipe from Hope's grandmother. The original meatballs were made with pork. This version contains tofu "meatballs," which are delicious, low-fat, and phytoestrogen rich. Escarole is a leafy green rich in folic acid and vitamin A, nutrients important for their antioxidant and cancer-prevention properties. Tip: *Turn the tofu meatballs gently. They have a tendency to crumble.*

Preparation: 20 minutes
Cooking: 30 minutes
Yield: 4 main-course servings

TOFU MEATBALLS

2 teaspoons olive oil

3 cloves garlic, peeled and sliced

1 medium onion, finely chopped

1 teaspoon dried basil

Sea salt to taste

⅓ cup flat-leaf parsley, finely chopped

12 ounces firm tofu, mashed

½ cup grated Romano cheese

1 cup breadcrumbs

1 egg

Black pepper to taste

2 tablespoons canola oil

REMAINING INGREDIENTS

2 teaspoons olive oil

3 cloves garlic, peeled and sliced

1½ pounds escarole, chopped, washed, and drained

10 cups hot vegetable broth (see page 124) or canned vegetable broth

⅓ pound cavatelli or other small pasta

4 teaspoons grated Romano cheese

1. To prepare the tofu meatballs, heat the olive oil in a skillet over low heat. Add the garlic and cook until soft and fragrant. Add the onion and basil to the skillet. Sprinkle the onion with sea salt and cook until it is soft, stirring occasionally. Add the parsley to the skillet.

2. Place the tofu in the work bowl of a food processor fitted with a metal blade. Add the onion mixture to the tofu. Add the Romano cheese, breadcrumbs, and egg. Process the ingredients until they are smooth. Season the mixture with sea salt and black pepper.

3. Form the tofu mixture into 16 tightly packed balls.

4. Heat 1 tablespoon of canola oil in a large skillet over high heat. When the oil is hot, carefully place 8 of the balls in it. Reduce the heat slightly and cook the tofu balls until they are golden on all sides. Repeat this procedure with the remaining oil and tofu balls.

5. To complete the soup, heat olive oil in a Dutch oven over low heat. Add the garlic to the pot and cook until soft and fragrant.

6. Raise the heat to high and add the escarole to the pot. Cook the escarole for 2 minutes, stirring often.

7. Add the broth to the pot and bring the soup to a boil. Add the pasta to the boiling stock and cook until tender.

8. Float the tofu balls into the soup. Season with sea salt and black pepper.

9. Ladle the soup into 4 bowls and garnish each portion with a sprinkling of Romano cheese. Accompany with crusty bread.

Vegetable-Beef Soup with Israeli Couscous

Preparation: 10 minutes
Cooking: 2 hours
Yield: 4 main-course
servings

This light, yet hearty vegetable and beef soup contains many vegetables rich in both antioxidants and fiber, all important in cancer prevention. As in the Asian tradition, the texture of the silken tofu contrasts well with the beef. Tip: *Be certain to use a piece of chuck in this recipe, not a piece of round. Chuck contains more connective tissue than round and, when cooked long and gently, will be fork-tender and delicious.*

1 tablespoon canola oil
1 pound chuck, well trimmed and cut into small cubes
Sea salt to taste
Black pepper to taste
4 cloves garlic, peeled and sliced
1 onion, peeled and diced
2 ribs celery, diced
3 medium carrots, peeled and diced
1 parsnip, peeled and diced
1 portobello mushroom, stemmed and diced
2 cups fresh chicken broth or 1 15-ounce can low-sodium
   chicken broth
4 cups cold water
12 ounces silken tofu, cut into small cubes
⅔ cup Israeli couscous
8 ounces fresh spinach, trimmed and chopped

1. Heat the canola oil in a Dutch oven over high heat. Sprinkle the meat with sea salt and black pepper. When the oil is hot, carefully place the meat in the pot in a single layer. Sear the meat until it is well browned, approximately 5 minutes, stirring 2 or 3 times.

2. Reduce the heat to low, remove the meat from the pot, and set aside. Add the garlic to the pot and cook for 30 seconds. Add the onion and a dash of sea salt. Cook the onion until soft, stirring often. Add the celery, carrots, parsnip, and mushroom to the pot. Return the meat to the pot.

3. Cover the pot and cook the ingredients for 10 minutes, stirring occasionally. Raise the heat to high and add the chicken broth and water. Bring the soup to a boil. As soon as it boils, reduce the heat to a low simmer. Skim the foam that rises to the surface of the soup and discard it. Stir the tofu into the soup.

4. Cover the pot and simmer the soup for 1½ hours. Remove the soup from the heat and stir in the couscous and spinach. Season with sea salt and black pepper. Cover the pot and allow the soup to rest for 10 minutes.

5. Ladle the soup into 4 large bowls and accompany with crusty bread and, if desired, a green salad.

Wakame Soup with Shiitake Mushrooms and Udon Noodles

Preparation: 15 minutes
Cooking: 35 minutes
Yield: 4 main-course servings

This Asian-inspired soup is light and delicious, yet filling enough to make a meal. The tofu is rich in phytoestrogens, and the wakame, a cultivated sea vegetable, is a great source of calcium. Tips: *Wakame is available in Asian markets and natural food stores. Dried shiitake mushrooms are widely available and are a better value than fresh ones. Also, their soaking liquid is a great addition to soups and sauces. If you can't locate udon noodles, linguine is a good substitute.*

1 ounce dried shiitake mushrooms, stems removed and discarded
1½ cups boiling water for mushrooms
Sea salt to taste
8 ounces udon noodles
2 teaspoons canola oil
3 cloves garlic, peeled and sliced
1 1-inch piece gingerroot, peeled and chopped
1 onion, peeled and diced
6 scallions, trimmed and sliced, white and green parts separated
1 carrot, peeled and diced
8 5-inch strips wakame, torn into 3 pieces each
9 cups vegetable broth (see page 124)

8 ounces silken tofu, cut into small cubes

2 tablespoons shoyu or tamari

½ cup cilantro, chopped

1. Place the mushrooms in a bowl. Pour the boiling water on them and allow to macerate for 20 minutes.

2. While the mushrooms are soaking, bring a pot of water to a boil. Add sea salt to the water, followed by the noodles. Cook the noodles until tender, approximately 4 minutes. Drain them and set aside.

3. Heat the oil in a Dutch oven over low heat. Add the garlic and gingerroot to the pot and cook until they are soft and fragrant.

4. Add the onion and the white parts of the scallions to the pot and cook until they begin to soften. Raise the heat slightly and add the carrot and wakame. Sprinkle the vegetables with sea salt.

5. Cover the pot and steam the vegetables for 5 minutes, stirring occasionally.

6. Drain the mushrooms and reserve their soaking water. Slice them and add them to the pot along with their soaking water.

7. Raise the heat to high and bring the liquid to a boil, reduce the heat, and simmer for 5 minutes.

8. Add the vegetable broth to the pot and bring the soup to a boil. Stir in the tofu. Reduce the heat to a simmer and cover the pot. Simmer for 20 minutes. Season with sea salt.

9. Divide the noodles among 4 large soup bowls. Ladle the soup into each bowl. Garnish each serving with the green parts of the scallions, shoyu, and cilantro.

Tempeh, Zucchini, and Beef Chili

Combining meat and soy is by no means a novel idea. It is a ubiquitous pairing in Asian cuisines. The tempeh in this beef chili adds a dose of phytoestrogens to a meal that the most die-hard meat-eater will love. To make a vegetarian version, eliminate the

Preparation: 30 minutes
Cooking: 2 hours
Yield: 6 main-course
servings

meat and add 2 cups of cooked bulgur during the last 15 minutes of cooking. Tips: *The chili can be prepared a day in advance and refrigerated. Reheat it gently to prevent from scorching. Also, it can be cooked in a slow (275°F) oven for 1 1/2 hours. As the recipe directs, finish the chili on the range.*

2 small dried chilies
2 cups water, boiling
2 tablespoons canola oil, divided
8 ounces beef chuck, trimmed and cut into ½-inch cubes
Sea salt to taste
Black pepper to taste
8 ounces tempeh, cut into small cubes
6 cloves garlic, peeled and sliced
1 onion, peeled and sliced
1 red bell pepper, cored and sliced
1 green bell pepper, cored and sliced
2 carrots, peeled and diced
1 zucchini, peeled and diced
1 tablespoon chili powder
1 teaspoon cumin
1 teaspoon dried oregano
2 cups chili-soaking water
1 15-ounce can red kidney beans, drained and rinsed
1 28-ounce can crushed tomatoes
4 ounces soy cheddar, grated or sliced

1. Place the dried chilies in a bowl and pour the boiling water on them. Allow them to macerate for 15 minutes. Drain them and reserve their soaking water.

2. Meanwhile, heat 1 tablespoon of the oil in a Dutch oven over high heat. Sprinkle the meat with sea salt and black pepper. When the oil is hot, carefully place the meat in the pot in a single layer. Sear the meat until well browned, approximately 5 minutes, turning 2 or 3 times. Add the tempeh to the pot and sear it as well until golden, approximately 3 minutes,

turning 2 or 3 times. Reduce the heat to low, remove the ingredients from the pot, and set aside.

3. Heat the remaining tablespoon of oil in the Dutch oven over low heat. Add the garlic and cook for 1 minute. Add the onion to the pot and a dash of sea salt. Cook the onion until soft, stirring it often.

4. Add the bell peppers, carrots, zucchini, chili powder, cumin, oregano, and the reserved meat and tempeh. Stir the ingredients, cover the pot, and steam the ingredients for 10 minutes, stirring them occasionally.

5. Raise the heat to high and add the reserved chili-soaking water, kidney beans, and crushed tomatoes to the pot. Bring to a boil, reduce the heat to a low simmer, cover the pot, and cook for 1½ hours.

6. Uncover the pot, raise the heat to medium, and simmer for 15 minutes longer, stirring occasionally. Season the chili with sea salt and black pepper.

7. Divide the chili among 6 large bowls and garnish each serving with soy cheddar.

Black Bean Soup with Lemon and Parsley

This slightly spicy black bean soup is refreshing with the tangy flavor of lemon and parsley. Black beans are a terrific source of fiber, important in the prevention of many cancers. This version is finished with pureed silken tofu in order to provide phytoestrogens. Tips: *Although we offer the alternative of using canned beans in many recipes throughout the book, this is a case where dried beans truly make a better soup. The soup can be made a day in advance. Heat it over low heat, adding water, if necessary, to thin it.*

Preparation: 20 minutes
Cooking: 1½ hours
Yield: 4 main-course servings

1 pound dried black turtle beans, picked over, rinsed, and
   soaked for eight hours
8 cups water
1 tablespoon olive oil
3 cloves garlic, peeled and sliced
1 onion, peeled and diced
1 jalapeño pepper, cored, seeded, and diced
2 carrots, peeled and diced
2 ribs celery, diced
Sea salt to taste
2 teaspoons ground coriander
2 teaspoons cumin powder
2 cups water
Bean cooking water
12 ounces silken tofu, chopped
½ cup flat-leaf parsley, chopped
Juice from one lemon
Black pepper to taste
4 scallions, thinly sliced

1. Place the beans in a Dutch oven and cover with the water. Bring the water to a boil. Reduce the heat and partly cover the pot. Simmer the beans until they are tender, approximately 1¼ hours. Drain the beans and reserve their cooking water.

2. While the beans are simmering, heat the olive oil in a skillet over low heat. Add the garlic to the oil and cook it until it is soft and fragrant. Add the onion to the skillet and cook until soft, stirring occasionally.

3. Add the jalapeño, carrots, celery, and a pinch of sea salt to the skillet. Cover the skillet and steam the vegetables for 8 minutes, stirring occasionally. Add the coriander and cumin to the vegetables.

4. Add the water to the skillet and bring to a boil. Reduce the heat and simmer for 5 minutes. Set the skillet aside.

5. In the work bowl of a food processor fitted with a metal

blade, puree half of the cooked beans with their cooking water and the tofu. Return the bean-tofu puree to the Dutch oven.

6. Stir the vegetables into the beans. Add the parsley and lemon juice to the soup. Season with sea salt and black pepper.

7. Divide the soup among 4 large bowls and garnish each serving with the scallions. Accompany with rustic bread and plain yogurt.

Chapter 12

Spreads and Sandwiches

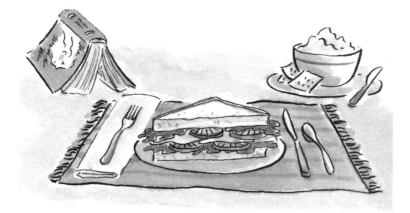

For a quick lunch, a light supper, a snack, or an appetizer, spreads and sandwiches are some of our favorite dishes. The spreads and sandwiches in this chapter range from the simple to the creative. Our delicious soy-based spreads and tofu sandwiches are nutritious and practical. Try the old standby, Egg Salad Sandwich, made with tofu mayonnaise, or the unique Tofu, Eggplant, and Swiss Chard Roll-Ups, balsamic-flavored vegetables and tofu spread with a basil pesto and rolled into a flour tortilla. Both are simple to prepare and phytoestrogen powerhouses. Our two soy-based burgers—Tofu, Spinach, and Shiitake and Tofu, White Bean, and Corn—may make you forget about fatty meat burgers forever.

Some of the other spreads in this chapter not only are wonderful on sandwiches but can be served as dips and pasta toppings as well. Next time you are entertaining or simply want to snack, try one of the traditional favorites—Guacamole, Hummus, or Baba Ghanoush, prepared our tofu-based way—bursting with flavor and texture and loaded with phytoestrogens. Or if you are craving pasta and don't want to fuss, toss hot cooked pasta with a bit of pasta-cooking water and our tofu-based Olive, Dried Tomato, and Basil Pesto.

Soy-based sandwiches and spreads are simple to prepare, versatile, and nutritious. Humble foods like tofu and soy beans make creative sandwiches and spreads. Most important, they are estrogenic feasts.

White Bean, Dried Tomato, and Balsamic Spread

Earthy, sweet, and tart, this spread is a great source of fiber and phytoestrogens. For a quick sandwich spread it on a bagel and top it with your favorite vegetables or top it with soy cheese and bake until the cheese melts.

Preparation: 15 minutes
Cooking: 0
Yield: 2 cups

½ **cup dried tomatoes**
1 **cup boiling water**
1 **15-ounce can navy beans, drained and rinsed**
1 **small clove garlic, peeled and minced**
1–2 **tablespoons top-quality balsamic vinegar**
6 **ounces silken tofu**
Sea salt to taste
Black pepper to taste

1. Place the tomatoes in a bowl. Pour the water on them and allow to soften for 10 minutes. Drain the tomatoes and set aside.

2. Combine the beans, garlic, vinegar, tofu, and tomatoes in a work bowl of a food processor fitted with a metal blade. Process the ingredients until a smooth spread forms. Season the spread with sea salt and black pepper.

3. Transfer the spread to a bowl and refrigerate until it is needed.

Tofu Parsley Hummus

Preparation: 10 minutes
Cooking: 0
Yield: 2 cups

Spread this creamy hummus on your favorite sandwich or stir it into hot pasta for a simple and delicious phytoestrogen- and fiber-rich meal. Tip: *The consistency of sesame tahini is similar to that of natural peanut butter—the oil tends to rise. Vigorously shaking the can is an efficient method for reincorporating the oil into the solids.*

1 15-ounce can chickpeas, drained and rinsed
1 small clove garlic, peeled and finely chopped
6 ounces silken tofu, chopped
¼ cup flat-leaf parsley, chopped
5 tablespoons sesame tahini
Juice from 1 lemon
Sea salt to taste
Black pepper to taste
Romaine leaves, washed and dried
1 large tomato, sliced
Bean sprouts

1. In the work bowl of a food processor fitted with a metal blade combine the chickpeas, garlic, tofu, parsley, tahini, and lemon juice. Process the ingredients until they are smooth. Season with sea salt and black pepper.

2. Serve the hummus spread on bagels with lettuce, tomatoes, and bean sprouts.

> **Tahini**
>
> Traditional Middle Eastern spreads, such as Baba Ghanoush (eggplant based) and Hummus (chickpea based), use sesame tahini as a main ingredient. Not to be confused with sesame butter, in which the seeds are roasted before being ground, tahini is made from crushed sesame seeds. It has a rich and creamy flavor and, like all pureed nuts and seeds, it is high in calories and fat. It is, though, a good source of protein and calcium. We find it adds richness to dressings, sauces, and chilled pasta salads.

Spicy Black Bean Hummus

Black beans make a unique hummus with a smooth consistency. Our spicy version is rich in fiber, calcium (from the tahini), and phytoestrogens. Serve it as a dip; spread it into burritos, quesadillas, or pitas; or toss it with hot pasta and your favorite vegetables.

Preparation: 10 minutes
Cooking: 0
Yield: 2 cups

1 15-ounce can black beans, drained and rinsed
1 small clove garlic, peeled and finely chopped
½ Scotch bonnet pepper, seeded and minced
6 ounces silken tofu, chopped
¼ cup fresh basil, chopped
4 tablespoons sesame tahini
Juice from 1½ lemons
Sea salt to taste
Black pepper to taste

1. In the work bowl of a food processor fitted with a metal blade combine the black beans, garlic, pepper, tofu, basil, tahini, and lemon juice. Process the ingredients until smooth. Season with sea salt and black pepper.

Baba Ghanoush

Preparation: 10 minutes
Cooking: 35 minutes
Yield: 4 servings

Sweet, smoky, and creamy, this Middle Eastern eggplant spread is a staple in our refrigerator. With silken tofu as a major ingredient, it is an excellent recipe to have in your repertoire. Serve it our favorite way—spread on chewy sesame bagels with a few leaves of arugula, sliced tomatoes, sea salt, and a drizzle of extra-virgin olive oil. Tip: *Italian eggplants are the top choice for this recipe. Since they are smaller than the ubiquitous large, purple variety, they do not take as long to cook, and, more important, they contain fewer seeds and are therefore less bitter.*

3 Italian eggplants (about 2 pounds)
1 small clove garlic, peeled and crushed
Juice from 1½ lemons
4 ounces silken tofu
4 tablespoons tahini
1 tablespoon olive oil
Sea salt to taste
Black pepper to taste
3 scallions, trimmed and thinly sliced

1. Heat the oven to 375°F. Place the eggplants on a heavy baking sheet and roast them until tender, approximately 35 minutes. Allow to cool. Remove the skin and transfer the pulp to a bowl. Discard the skin.

2. Meanwhile, in the work bowl of a food processor fitted with a metal blade, combine the garlic, lemon juice, tofu, tahini, and olive oil. Process the ingredients until smooth. Add the eggplant to the bowl and process until well combined.

3. Season with sea salt and black pepper. Transfer the spread to a bowl and garnish with the scallions.

Guacamole

Rich-tasting avocados and silken tofu have an affinity for each other. In this recipe they are combined to make a creamy phyto-estrogen-rich guacamole. Use it as a dip for chips or spread it on a sandwich or in a burrito. Tip: *This is a mellow-flavored version. If you prefer a spicier guacamole, add a diced hot pepper or a few additional shakes of hot pepper sauce.*

Preparation: 10 minutes
Cooking: 0
Yield: 2 cups

6 ounces silken tofu
2 ripe avocados, halved and pitted
Juice from 1 large lemon
4 scallions, trimmed and thinly sliced
1 large tomato, diced
1 very small clove garlic, crushed or minced
Dash of hot-pepper sauce
Sea salt to taste
Black pepper to taste

1. Place the tofu in the work bowl of a food processor fitted with a metal blade. Puree the tofu and set it aside.

2. Scoop the avocados into a bowl. Add the lemon juice and with a fork mash the avocados coarsely.

3. Stir in the scallions, tomato, and garlic. Add the hot-pepper sauce and stir in the tofu. Season with sea salt and black pepper.

4. Serve the guacamole at room temperature within 3 hours.

Olive, Dried Tomato, and Basil Pesto

Use this intensely flavored pesto as a dip or a sandwich spread or toss it with hot pasta. No one needs to know that it contains silken tofu. Tip: *When seasoning the pesto, keep in mind that both olives and sun-dried tomatoes tend to be salty.*

Preparation: 20 minutes
Cooking: 0
Yield: 1½ cups

1 cup boiling water
1 cup sun-dried tomatoes
1⅓ cups fresh basil
16 Gaeta or 12 Kalamata olives, pitted and chopped
2 cloves garlic, peeled and chopped
2 tablespoons pine nuts
4 ounces silken tofu
2 tablespoons olive oil
4 tablespoons grated Parmesan or Romano cheese
Sea salt to taste
Black pepper to taste

1. Pour the water on the sun-dried tomatoes and allow them to soften, approximately 15 minutes.

2. While the tomatoes are softening, place the basil, olives, garlic, pine nuts, and tofu in the work bowl of a food processor fitted with a metal blade.

3. When the tomatoes are soft, drain them. Reserve their soaking water for another use. Coarsely chop them and add them to the work bowl.

4. Turn the machine on and drizzle in the olive oil. Process until a smooth paste forms. Stir in the Parmesan cheese. Season with sea salt and black pepper.

5. Transfer the pesto to a bowl and cover tightly. It will keep for 1 day in the refrigerator.

Broccoli–Basil Pesto

Preparation: 5 minutes
Cooking: 5 minutes
Yield: 2 cups

Besides being a key ingredient in Sue Salem's Marinated Tofu Sandwich (see page 150), this pesto is also wonderful tossed with hot pasta or as part of the filling for a burrito. It is rich in phytoestrogens and antioxidants. Tip: It will be necessary to turn your food processor off and push the ingredients back toward the blade several times.

1½ cups water

Sea salt to taste

1 pound broccoli, trimmed, stems peeled and sliced and
    florets separated

½ cup fresh basil

4 ounces silken tofu

3 tablespoons pine nuts

1 small clove garlic, peeled and minced

¼ cup grated Parmesan cheese

Black pepper to taste

1. Bring the water to a boil in a Dutch oven. Add a dash of sea salt to the water, followed by the broccoli. Cover the pot and steam the broccoli until it is just tender, approximately 4 minutes.

2. Drain the broccoli and spray with cold water. Squeeze the broccoli firmly to remove any excess water.

3. Transfer the broccoli to the work bowl of a food processor. Add the basil, tofu, pine nuts, and garlic to the bowl. Process until a smooth pesto forms, stopping the machine several times to scrape the ingredients in the bowl back toward the blade.

4. Transfer the pesto to a bowl and stir in the Parmesan cheese. Season with sea salt and black pepper. Cover the bowl. The pesto will keep in the refrigerator for 2 days.

Spinach–Artichoke Spread

This recipe was adapted from a mayonnaise-based artichoke dip recipe. By replacing the mayonnaise with silken tofu, our version is significantly lower in fat than other versions and a great source of phytoestrogens.

Preparation: 10 minutes
Cooking: 0
Yield: 2 cups

3 cups fresh spinach, trimmed, washed, and spun dry
1 14-ounce jar artichoke hearts, drained and rinsed
1 clove garlic, peeled and minced
Juice from ½ lemon
1 teaspoon Dijon mustard
6 ounces silken tofu
⅓ cup grated Parmesan cheese
Sea salt to taste
Black pepper to taste

1. Combine the spinach, artichoke hearts, garlic, lemon juice, Dijon mustard, and tofu in the work bowl of a food processor fitted with a metal blade. Turn the machine on and blend until a smooth spread forms.

2. Stir the Parmesan cheese into the spread and season with sea salt and black pepper. Either use the spread at once or transfer it to a sealed container and refrigerate. It will keep for 2 days.

Arugula and Cilantro Pesto

Preparation: 10 minutes
Cooking: 0
Yield: 1½ cups

This pesto is rich in phytoestrogens since it contains silken tofu. Try it as a spread on a sandwich or crusty bread for an appetizer, or toss it with pasta for a quick meal. Tip: Arugula tends to be sandy. Wash it in 2 or 3 changes of water.

1½ cups arugula, thoroughly washed and dried
1 cup cilantro
1 clove garlic, peeled and chopped
3 tablespoons pine nuts
4 ounces silken tofu
2 tablespoons extra-virgin olive oil
4 tablespoons grated Parmesan cheese
Sea salt to taste
Black pepper to taste

1. Combine the arugula, cilantro, garlic, pine nuts, and tofu in the work bowl of a food processor fitted with a metal blade.

2. Turn the machine on and drizzle in the olive oil. Process until a smooth paste forms. Stir in the Parmesan cheese and season with sea salt and black pepper.

3. Transfer the pesto to a bowl and cover tightly. It will keep for 1 day in the refrigerator.

Polenta Sandwiches

These open-faced sandwiches use baked polenta squares instead of bread. The toppings are suggestions. Use your imagination and any bits and pieces in your refrigerator to come up with your own delectable sandwiches. Tip: *The polenta can be made a day in advance and refrigerated in the baking pan.*

Preparation: 50 minutes
Cooking: 10 minutes
Yield: 4 sandwiches

1 recipe for Polenta (without the Blue Castello) (see page 272)

TOPPINGS
Italian style: Fresh tomatoes, basil, extra-virgin olive oil, and soy mozzarella
Greek style: Sautéed spinach and feta cheese
Mexican style: Pureed spicy soybeans, salsa, cilantro, and soy cheddar

1. Prepare the polenta according to the recipe on page 000. Spread the polenta into a lightly oiled 8 x 8–inch baking pan. Allow the polenta to cool. Heat the oven to 375°F.

2. When the polenta is cool, cut it into 8 squares. Transfer 4 of the polenta squares to a baking sheet. Place an equal amount of topping on each. Top each square with another piece of polenta to form sandwiches.

3. Transfer the tray to the oven and bake the sandwiches until they are hot, approximately 10 minutes.

Sue Salem's Marinated Tofu Sandwich

Preparation: 10 minutes
Marinating: 1 to 2 hours
Cooking: 20 minutes
Yield: 4 main-course servings

One of Hope's patients suggested this recipe; it is an incredibly healthful sandwich. The tofu takes on the flavor of the marinade, and the broccoli-basil pesto adds moisture and a fresh flavor. It is phytoestrogen and calcium-rich from the tofu and the pesto, which contains silken tofu. Tips: *The marinade detailed here is one suggestion. This recipe is meant to be flexible; use your imagination and vary the ingredients to suit your taste. Also, the Broccoli-Basil Pesto can be prepared a day in advance and refrigerated.*

½ cup orange juice
3 tablespoons balsamic vinegar
1 clove garlic, peeled and minced
⅓ cup fresh basil, snipped
Sea salt to taste
Black pepper to taste
1 pound extra-firm tofu, sliced into 4 rectangles
8 slices multigrain bread, toasted
4 tablespoons Broccoli-Basil Pesto (see page 146)
1 tomato, sliced
2 ounces alfalfa sprouts
6 ounces fresh spinach leaves

1. Combine the orange juice, vinegar, garlic, basil, sea salt, and black pepper in a shallow, nonmetal pan. Place the tofu into the pan and spoon some of the marinade onto it. Marinate the tofu for 1 to 2 hours, turning it occasionally.

2. Heat the oven to 375°F. Transfer the tofu to a baking sheet. Spoon 1 tablespoon of the marinade onto each piece of tofu and bake the tofu until it is golden, approximately 15 minutes. Remove the tofu from the oven and set aside.

3. To assemble a sandwich, take 2 slices of bread and spread 1 tablespoon of Broccoli-Basil Pesto onto each slice. Place a piece of tofu on one of the slices and top with a slice of

tomato, sprouts, and spinach. Place the other slice of bread on top and cut the sandwich in half.

4. Repeat the procedure with the remaining ingredients. If desired, accompany with baked potato chips.

Marinating Tofu

The bland flavor of tofu makes it an ideal food to marinate. Strongly flavored vinegars, fermented soy products (miso and shoyu), and plenty of ginger, garlic, and onions will transform an ordinary block of tofu into something special.

Slice tofu into ½-inch-thick blocks and marinate them in a shallow pan for an hour or two. Turn the tofu occasionally with a spatula carefully to prevent the blocks from breaking. Marinated tofu can be grilled, baked, and pan cooked.

Tofu, Eggplant, and Swiss Chard Roll-Ups with Basil Pesto

Roll-up sandwiches are becoming increasingly popular. They allow you to use ingredients that would make a traditional sandwich fall apart. In this version the tofu, eggplant, and Swiss chard are rolled with basil pesto (with silken tofu) and soy jack cheese, making this meal rich in phytoestrogens. Tip: *This recipe requires preparing a basil pesto with silken tofu, but feel free to use any of the spreads found at the beginning of this chapter. The pesto in this recipe is also wonderful tossed with pasta.*

Preparation: 15 minutes
Cooking: 40 minutes
Yield: 4 main-course servings

2½ cups water

Sea salt to taste

1 cup short-grain brown rice

4 cups fresh basil leaves

1 clove garlic, peeled and minced

⅓ cup pine nuts

6 ounces silken tofu

⅓ cup grated Parmesan cheese

Black pepper to taste

2 tablespoons olive oil, divided

1 pound firm tofu, cut into small cubes

2 Japanese or Italian eggplants, cubed

4 tablespoons top-quality balsamic vinegar

5 cloves garlic, peeled and sliced

1½ pounds Swiss chard, trimmed, chopped, washed, and drained

4 ounces soy jack cheese, sliced or grated

4 large flour tortillas

1. Bring the water to a boil in a medium saucepan. Add sea salt to the water and stir in the rice. Bring the water back to a boil, cover the pot, leaving the lid slightly ajar, reduce the heat, and simmer until the water is absorbed, approximately 40 minutes.

2. While the rice is cooking, prepare the pesto by combining the basil, garlic, pine nuts, and silken tofu in the work bowl of a food processor fitted with a metal blade. Puree the ingredients until a smooth pesto forms. Stir in the Parmesan cheese and season with sea salt and black pepper. Set the pesto aside.

3. Heat 1 tablespoon of the olive oil in a wok over high heat. When the oil is hot, add the firm tofu and eggplant to the wok. Cook until golden, stirring 3 or 4 times. Add the vinegar to the wok and cook for 30 seconds more. Transfer to a plate.

4. Heat the remaining olive oil in the wok over medium heat. Add the garlic to the wok and cook for 1 minute. Raise the heat to high and add the chard to the wok. Stir the chard

and cook for 1 minute. Reduce the heat to medium, cover the pan, and steam the chard until tender. If necessary, add water to the chard to prevent it from burning. Stir the tofu-eggplant mixture into the chard and remove the pan from the heat.

5. To assemble the sandwiches, divide the cheese among the tortillas. Melt the cheese either in a microwave or in an oven at low heat. Spread a portion of the pesto on each tortilla and add a large spoonful of the rice and vegetable-tofu mixture. Roll the sandwiches and serve them at once.

Egg Salad Sandwich

Mayonnaise and eggs are foods one should not eat regularly because of the saturated fat and cholesterol. But with a tofu-based dressing and only one-half of a yolk per serving, it is fine to indulge in this egg salad sandwich. Tip: *Use the tofu-mayonnaise as a spread for other sandwiches.*

Preparation: 10 minutes
Cooking: 10 minutes
Yield: 4 main-course dish servings

DRESSING
4 ounces plain nonfat yogurt
1 tablespoon sugar
1 small clove garlic, peeled and minced
1 tablespoon tahini
1 teaspoon Dijon mustard
1 tablespoon cider vinegar
4 ounces silken tofu
Sea salt to taste
Black pepper to taste

REMAINING INGREDIENTS
2 hard-cooked eggs
8 hard-cooked egg whites
8 slices rustic bread or 4 bagels, sliced
Lettuce leaves
Tomato slices

1. Combine the yogurt, sugar, garlic, tahini, mustard, vinegar, and tofu in the work bowl of a food processor fitted with a metal blade. Process until a creamy dressing forms. Season with sea salt and black pepper. Set aside.

2. Coarsely chop the eggs and egg whites and place them in a bowl. Stir in the dressing and season with sea salt and black pepper.

3. Using the bread or bagels, make 4 sandwiches. Add lettuce and tomato to each sandwich. Accompany with a mesclun salad.

Udon Noodle Roll-Ups

Preparation: 15 minutes
Cooking: 15 minutes
Yield: 4 main-course servings

It is fun to be creative with rolled sandwiches. In this version udon noodles, tofu, and an array of vegetables are rolled into a whole-wheat flour tortilla, making this roll-up rich in phytoestrogens, fiber, and antioxidants. Tips: *Make a double recipe; have the filling as a noodle dish one day and a roll-up the next. If you can't locate udon noodles, substitute whole-wheat spaghetti or linguine.*

SAUCE

   1 teaspoon sesame oil

   2 tablespoons ketchup

   1 tablespoon Dijon mustard

   2 tablespoons cider vinegar

   3 tablespoons shoyu or tamari

   3 tablespoons oyster sauce

   1 cup low-sodium chicken broth

   1 teaspoon sugar

REMAINING INGREDIENTS

   Sea salt to taste

   8 ounces brown-rice udon noodles

   1 cup water

   1 pound broccoli, trimmed, stems trimmed and cut into matchsticks, florets cut into 2-inch pieces

2 tablespoons canola oil, divided

1 pound firm tofu, sliced into small cubes

1 1-inch piece gingerroot, peeled and minced

3 cloves garlic, peeled and sliced

1 red bell pepper, cored and thinly sliced

8 ounces bok choy, trimmed, stems sliced diagonally into ¾-inch-thick pieces and leaves coarsely chopped and separated

4 12-inch whole-wheat flour tortillas, warmed

1. Make the sauce by whisking together the sesame oil, ketchup, Dijon mustard, vinegar, shoyu, oyster sauce, broth, and sugar.

2. Meanwhile, bring a large pot of water to a boil. Add sea salt to the water, followed by the noodles. Cook the noodles until tender. Drain and set them aside.

3. Place the water in a Dutch oven and bring to a boil. Add a dash of sea salt to the water. Add the broccoli to the pot and cover it. Steam the broccoli for 5 minutes. Drain and cool it under cold running water. Set the broccoli aside.

4. Heat 1 tablespoon of the oil in a wok over high heat. When the oil is hot, add the tofu to the wok. Cook the tofu until golden, stirring several times. Transfer the tofu to a plate and set aside.

5. Heat the remaining oil in the wok over high heat. When the oil is hot, add the gingerroot and garlic to the wok, and cook for 30 seconds. Add the bell pepper and bok choy stems to the wok. Cook the vegetables until they begin to soften, stirring often. Add the bok choy leaves to the wok and cook for 30 seconds, stirring constantly.

6. Add the broccoli and tofu to the wok. Cook them until they are hot, stirring often. Whisk the sauce and pour it into the wok. Add the noodles to the wok. Cook the pasta and sauce together for 1 minute. Remove the wok from the heat.

7. Divide the noodles among the 4 flour tortillas. Roll each tortilla into a tube. Serve the roll-ups hot or at room temperature.

Tempeh and Mozzarella Melts with a Honey–Mustard Sauce

Preparation: 5 minutes
Cooking: 15 minutes
Yield: 4 main-course servings

Who needs meat as a sandwich filling when you can have tempeh? In this recipe hearty tempeh is brushed with a balsamic vinaigrette, baked, and topped with soy mozzarella. A honey-mustard sauce provides a lot of flavor with no fat. These phytoestrogen-rich sandwiches are also a great source of calcium from the cheese and Romaine lettuce.

1 tablespoon olive oil
1 tablespoon balsamic vinegar
2 teaspoons plus 1 tablespoon Dijon mustard
8 ounces tempeh
Sea salt to taste
Black pepper to taste
3 tablespoons honey
2 ounces soy mozzarella, sliced or grated
4 English muffins, toasted
4 large romaine lettuce leaves

1. Heat the oven to 400°F. In a small bowl whisk the olive oil, vinegar, and 2 teaspoons of the Dijon mustard.

2. Cut the tempeh in half, then slice each piece in half through the middle to make it half as thick as it was. You now have 4 pieces. Sprinkle the tempeh with sea salt and black pepper.

3. Place the tempeh on a baking tray. Brush the top of each piece with the olive oil mixture.

4. Place the tray in the oven and bake the tempeh pieces until crisp and golden, approximately 12 minutes.

5. Meanwhile, to make the honey-mustard sauce, whisk together the remaining tablespoon of mustard and the honey. Set aside.

6. When the tempeh slices are done, place an equal amount of mozzarella on each. Bake until the cheese melts, approximately 3 minutes.

7. To make the sandwiches, place a piece of tempeh on one half of an English muffin. Spoon on a portion of the honey-mustard sauce and a romaine lettuce leaf. Top the sandwich with the other half of the English muffin. Repeat the procedure with the remaining ingredients. Serve at once.

Sesame Tempeh Burgers with a Tahini-Yogurt Sauce

These unique, Asian-flavored burgers substitute tempeh for meat or poultry. The sandwiches have 3 sources of phytoestrogens: tempeh, tofu, and miso. Romaine lettuce, yogurt, and tahini are good sources of calcium.

Preparation: 5 minutes
Cooking: 15 minutes
Yield: 4 main-course servings

1 tablespoon sesame oil
2 tablespoons shoyu or tamari
1 teaspoon miso
1 teaspoon Dijon mustard
8 ounces tempeh
Sea salt to taste
Black pepper to taste
8 ounces nonfat plain yogurt
3 ounces silken tofu, pureed
1 small clove garlic, peeled and minced
1 scallion, trimmed and thinly sliced
1 tablespoon sesame tahini
4 sandwich buns
4 large romaine lettuce leaves
4 slices tomato

1. Heat the oven to 400°F. In a small bowl whisk the sesame oil, shoyu, miso, and Dijon mustard.

2. Cut the tempeh in half; then slice each section in half through the middle to make it half as thick. You now have 4 pieces. Sprinkle the tempeh with sea salt and black pepper.

3. Place the tempeh on a baking tray. Brush the top of each piece with the sesame oil mixture.

4. Place the tray in the oven and bake the tempeh pieces until crisp and golden, approximately 12 minutes.

5. Meanwhile, to make the yogurt-tahini sauce, whisk together the yogurt, tofu, garlic, scallion, and tahini. Set aside.

6. To make the sandwiches, place a piece of tempeh on one half of a sandwich bun. Spoon on a portion of the yogurt-tahini sauce. Top the sandwich with a romaine lettuce leaf, a slice of tomato, and the other half of the bun. Repeat the procedure with the remaining ingredients. Serve at once.

Tempeh and Cheese Sandwiches with Peppers and Onions

Preparation: 10 minutes
Cooking: 30 minutes
Yield: 4 main-course servings

You won't find this version of the popular steak and cheese sandwich at your neighborhood pizza shop. With plenty of flavor from slowly cooked peppers and onions and plenty of phytoestrogen from the tempeh and soy cheddar, it is sure to become a favorite of yours. Tip: *The tempeh, peppers, and onions can be cooked a day in advance and refrigerated. Slowly heat the ingredients in a pan the following day.*

2 tomatoes, diced
2 tablespoons olive oil, divided
Sea salt to taste
Black pepper to taste

2 large onions, peeled and thinly sliced

1 large red bell pepper, seeded and thinly sliced

1 large green bell pepper, seeded and thinly sliced

8 ounces tempeh, cubed

1 tablespoon sugar

4 ounces soy cheddar

4 large flour tortillas

1. Place the tomatoes in a bowl. Drizzle with 1 tablespoon of the oil. Season with sea salt and black pepper. Set the tomatoes aside.

2. Heat the remaining tablespoon of olive oil in a Dutch oven over high heat. When the oil is hot, add the onions to the pot. Cook them for 1 minute, stirring constantly. Add the bell peppers to the pot and cook for another minute, stirring constantly. Add the tempeh to the pot and reduce the heat to low. Season with sea salt and black pepper.

3. Cover the pot and cook the ingredients for 15 minutes, stirring occasionally. Uncover the pot, add the sugar, and cook for another 10 minutes, stirring occasionally.

4. Divide the cheese among the 4 tortillas. Melt the cheese in a microwave or oven at low heat. Divide the filling among the 4 tortillas. Divide the tomatoes among the 4 sandwiches. Roll the sandwiches and serve immediately.

Tofu, Spinach, and Shiitake Burgers

Tofu is combined with spinach and shiitake mushrooms to create these robustly flavored burgers. With large amounts of calcium, phytoestrogens, and fiber and the same high-quality protein that a meat-based burger contains, these soy-based burgers are supernutritious. Tips: *The mix can be prepared a day in advance without the egg. Don't discard the mushroom-soaking water. It can be frozen for future use in a soup or sauce.*

Preparation: 15 minutes
Cooking: 10 minutes
Yield: 4 main-course servings

1 cup dried shiitake mushrooms, stems removed and
   discarded
1½ cups boiling water
2 teaspoons olive oil
4 cloves garlic, peeled and thinly sliced
1 onion, peeled and diced
8 ounces frozen chopped spinach, thawed
Sea salt to taste
Black pepper to taste
12 ounces firm tofu, crumbled
1 cup breadcrumbs
1 egg
1 tablespoon canola oil
2 ounces soy cheddar, sliced or grated
4 whole-grain sandwich buns
Tomato slices

1. Heat the oven to 400°F. Place the mushrooms in a bowl. Pour the water on them and allow to soften for 10 minutes. Drain them and set aside.

2. Heat the olive oil in a skillet over low heat. Add the garlic to the pan and cook until soft, stirring occasionally. Add the onion to the pan and cook until soft, stirring occasionally.

3. Squeeze as much moisture out of the spinach as possible and add it to the pan. Cook the ingredients for another three minutes, stirring occasionally. Season with sea salt and black pepper.

4. Transfer the ingredients to the work bowl of a food processor fitted with a metal blade. Add the tofu, breadcrumbs, egg, and mushrooms to the bowl. Turn the machine on and process the ingredients until well combined. It may be necessary to turn off the machine and scrape the ingredients back toward the blade.

5. Form the tofu mixture into 4 tightly packed balls. Form the balls into patties. Place the oil on a baking tray and place the tray in the oven for 3 minutes.

6. Remove the tray from the oven and place the patties on the tray. Bake until they are brown and crisp, approximately 10 minutes, turning them once. During the last 2 minutes, place an equal portion of cheese on each.

7. Divide the burgers among the 4 buns. Divide the tomato slices among the burgers and serve at once.

Tofu, White Bean, and Corn Burgers

Earthy and sweet tasting, these burgers provide plenty of phyto-estrogens from the tofu and a triple dose of fiber from the beans, corn, and tofu. Tip: *The mix can be prepared a day in advance without the egg.*

Preparation: 15 minutes
Cooking: 10 minutes
Yield: 4 main-course servings

½ cup dried tomatoes
1 cup boiling water
2 teaspoons olive oil
4 cloves garlic, peeled and thinly sliced
1 onion, peeled and diced
1 cup frozen corn
½ cup flat-leaf parsley, coarsely chopped
Sea salt to taste
Black pepper to taste
12 ounces firm tofu, crumbled
1 cup canned Great Northern beans, drained and rinsed
½ cup breadcrumbs
1 egg
1 tablespoon canola oil
2 ounces soy cheddar, sliced or grated
4 whole-grain sandwich buns
Tomato slices
Romaine lettuce leaves

1. Heat the oven to 400°F. Place the tomatoes in a bowl. Pour the water on them and allow to soften for 10 minutes. Drain and set aside.

2. Heat the olive oil in a skillet over low heat. Add the garlic to the pan and cook it until soft, stirring occasionally. Add the onion to the pan and cook until soft, stirring occasionally.

3. Add the corn and parsley to the pan. Cook the ingredients for another three minutes, stirring occasionally. Season with sea salt and black pepper.

4. Transfer the ingredients to the work bowl of a food processor fitted with a metal blade. Add the tofu, beans, breadcrumbs, egg, and tomatoes to the bowl. Turn the machine on and process the ingredients until well combined. It may be necessary to turn off the machine and scrape the ingredients back toward the blade.

5. Form the tofu mixture into 4 tightly packed balls. Form the balls into patties. Place the oil on a baking tray and place the tray in the oven for 3 minutes.

6. Remove the tray from the oven and place the patties on the tray. Bake the patties until browned and crisp, approximately 10 minutes, turning them once. During the last 2 minutes, place an equal portion of cheese on each.

7. Divide the burgers among the 4 buns. Divide the tomato slices and lettuce leaves among the burgers and serve at once.

Chapter 13

Salads

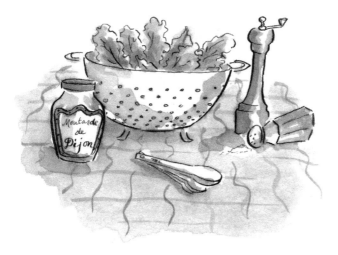

Whether you like your salads the traditional American way, at the beginning of the meal, or if you prefer them the way the Italians do, at the end, as long as you avoid fat-laden dressings, salads offer an abundance of nutrition and are a creative way to introduce soy into your diet. If you are like us, to avoid excess fat calories you probably eat your salads with a minimal amount of dressing. When they contain a tofu-based dressing, you can wave goodbye to dry salads forever. Well-coated greens translate into a greater amount of phytoestrogens in every forkful.

When it comes to soy-based salad dressing ingredients, silken tofu gets top billing. When pureed in a blender, silken tofu provides the base from which many delectable dressings can be prepared. Pureed tofu dressings have an affinity for crisp greens like romaine lettuce, endive, and radicchio, hearty vegetables like portobello mushrooms, and intensely flavored ingredients, such as lemon, balsamic vinegar, and tahini.

The salads in this chapter range from a Romaine and Radicchio Salad with Orange and Almonds to a main-dish salad of Romaine Lettuce with Garlicky Beef and Creamy Avocado Dressing. Both are wonderfully creamy and crisp with silken tofu as the main ingredient. Both are low in fat and provide an abundance of phytoestrogens and calcium. We also have included several lightly dressed and calcium-rich romaine salads for those times when you crave an olive oil–based dressing.

Whether served as a side dish or a main course, green salads with creamy tofu dressings are a delicious and low-fat way to get an abundance of soy and calcium into your diet.

Romaine Lettuce Salad with a Sesame-Garlic Dressing

Preparation: 10 minutes
Cooking: 0
Yield: 4 side-dish servings

Romaine lettuce is an excellent source of calcium. The base of the sesame-garlic dressing is silken tofu, not oil, so you can use more and still keep the fat content low and the phytoestrogen content high. Tips: The dressing can be prepared up to 3 days in advance and refrigerated. Whisk it before using. Also, if your cucumber is waxed, peel it.

DRESSING

4 ounces silken tofu
2 tablespoons sesame tahini
1 tablespoon dark miso
3 tablespoons cider vinegar
1 small garlic clove, peeled and crushed
1 tablespoon honey

Sea salt to taste
Black pepper to taste

SALAD
  1 head romaine lettuce, torn, washed, and spun dry
  2 tomatoes, cored and sliced into wedges
  1 cucumber, peeled, seeded, and sliced
  8 Kalamata olives, pitted and chopped
  2 ounces feta cheese, crumbled
  ¼ cup soy nuts

1. To prepare the dressing, combine the tofu, tahini, miso, vinegar, garlic, and honey in the work bowl of a food processor fitted with a metal blade. Process the ingredients until smooth. Transfer the dressing to a bowl and season with sea salt and black pepper. Set the dressing aside.

2. Place the romaine lettuce in a large bowl. Pour the dressing on the lettuce and toss well. Scatter on the tomatoes and the cucumber. Sprinkle with olives, feta cheese, and soy nuts.

3. Divide the salad among 4 bowls and serve at once.

Salad Preparation

To prepare great salads, use impeccable greens that have been washed, dried, and dressed carefully. First, fill a sink with very cold water. Tear or cut your greens with a sharp knife and place them in the water. Briefly swirl through the water and then drain. Place the greens in a salad spinner and spin until dry. Transfer to a bowl and cover with a dry dish towel. Refrigerate them until serving time. Just before serving, dress the salad with a room-temperature dressing. A warm dressing coats the greens more thoroughly than a chilled one does. If your salad contains ingredients other than greens, toss the greens with half of the dressing first, then add the other ingredients and toss with the remaining dressing.

Romaine Salad with Garlic Croutons and Balsamic Vinegar

Preparation: 10 minutes
Cooking: 15 minutes (croutons)
Yield: 4 side-dish servings

At first glance you may not realize that this is a calcium-rich salad. Romaine lettuce is a good source of calcium, while Parmesan cheese contains more calcium than do most hard cheeses. Tip: Save leftover pieces of rustic bread to make the garlic croutons. They can be prepared several days in advance. Wrap them tightly and freeze them. Thaw them for 30 minutes at room temperature before preparing the salad.

CROUTONS

1 12-inch-long loaf rustic bread
3 cloves garlic, peeled
2 tablespoon extra-virgin olive oil

DRESSING

2 tablespoons extra-virgin olive oil
2 tablespoons top-quality balsamic vinegar
1 tablespoon Dijon mustard
Sea salt to taste
Black pepper to taste

SALAD

1 large head romaine lettuce, trimmed, torn, washed, and thoroughly dried
4 ounces grated Parmesan cheese

1. Heat the oven to 400°F. Cut the bread in half lengthwise. Rub the garlic cloves on the inside of the bread. Drizzle the inside of the bread with 2 tablespoons of olive oil. Cut the bread into cubes and place on a baking tray. Bake the bread cubes until crisp, approximately 10 minutes. Remove from the oven and allow to cool.

2. Meanwhile, make the dressing by whisking together the

olive oil, balsamic vinegar, and Dijon mustard. Season with sea salt and black pepper.

3. Place the lettuce in a large bowl and pour the dressing on it. Add the croutons to the bowl and toss the salad well. Add the Parmesan cheese to the salad and toss once more.

4. Divide the salad among four chilled plates and serve at once.

Romaine Lettuce Salad with Caramelized Pears and Blue Cheese

This calcium-rich salad is one of our favorites. Caramelized pears are sweet and tender and provide a perfect contrast to the creamy blue cheese and crisp romaine lettuce. The blend of tastes and textures is delectable. Tip: *The pears can be cooked a day in advance and refrigerated. Bring them to room temperature before preparing the salad.*

Preparation: 10 minutes
Cooking: 20 minutes (pears)
Yield: 4 side-dish servings

SALAD

1 large head romaine lettuce, trimmed, torn, washed, and thoroughly dried
2 teaspoons canola oil
2 medium Bosc pears, scrubbed and thinly sliced
⅓ cup pecans, coarsely chopped
Sea salt to taste
2 ounces Blue Castello (or a similar creamy blue)

DRESSING

2 tablespoons extra-virgin olive oil
½ teaspoon Dijon mustard
2 tablespoons top-quality balsamic vinegar
Sea salt to taste
Black pepper to taste

1. Place the lettuce in a large salad bowl and refrigerate. Heat the canola oil in a medium-sized skillet over high heat. Add the pears to the skillet and reduce heat to low. Cook the pears until golden brown and sweet, stirring occasionally. Remove from the pan and allow to cool.

2. While the pears are caramelizing, place the pecans in a small skillet and sprinkle with sea salt. Toast over low heat, stirring often, until they are fragrant and no longer raw tasting. Set aside.

3. To make the dressing, whisk together the olive oil, mustard, and vinegar in a bowl until they emulsify. Season with sea salt and black pepper.

4. To assemble the salad, toss the lettuce with the pears, pecans, and dressing. Garnish with the Blue Castello. Divide the salad among four plates and serve at once.

Romaine Lettuce Salad with Crisp Vegetables, Blue Cheese, and Balsamic Vinegar

Preparation: 10 minutes
Cooking: 0
Yield: 4 side-dish servings

Blue cheese and balsamic vinegar have an affinity for each other. Unlike a traditional blue cheese dressing, this one is based upon silken tofu instead of oil, making it low in fat and rich in phytoestrogens. Tip: *Be certain to use only a small clove of garlic in this recipe. Too much raw garlic will overpower the other flavors in the salad.*

DRESSING

3 ounces crumbled blue cheese
6 ounces silken tofu
3 tablespoons top-quality balsamic vinegar
1 very small clove garlic, peeled and minced
⅓ cup fresh basil

4 tablespoons water
Sea salt to taste
Black pepper to taste

SALAD

1 head romaine lettuce, trimmed, torn, washed, and spun dry
1 head radicchio, trimmed and sliced
1 Belgian endive, trimmed and sliced
1 cucumber, peeled, seeded, and sliced
1 tomato, sliced into wedges

1. Place the blue cheese, tofu, vinegar, garlic, basil, and water in the work bowl of a food processor fitted with a metal blade. Process the ingredients until a smooth dressing forms. Season with sea salt and black pepper. Set aside.

2. Combine the romaine lettuce, radicchio, endive, and cucumber in a large salad bowl. Pour the dressing on the salad and toss well. Garnish the salad with the tomato wedges.

3. Divide the salad among 4 plates and serve immediately.

Radicchio

Ruby-colored radicchio is an endive that is delectable in a number of ways. Its crisp texture and peppery flavor make it ideal to combine with milder lettuces and a balsamic vinaigrette. It is a wonderful addition to a pasta dish. It doesn't need much cooking; add it to the sauce just before you stir in the pasta. The heat from the pasta will wilt it slightly, leaving the dish with a pleasant crunch. Radicchio is at its tastiest, though, when it is grilled (see recipe on page 217). The direct heat adds a hint of sweetness that other cooking methods don't produce.

Romaine and Mesclun Salad with a Lemon–Poppy Seed Dressing

Preparation: 10 minutes
Cooking: 10 minutes (croutons)
Yield: 4 side-dish servings

Silken tofu is the base for this slightly sweet yet citrusy dressing, making it rich in phytoestrogens yet low in fat. The blend of flavors in the mesclun lettuces and the romaine lettuce make this salad a wonderful contrast of tastes.

DRESSING

¼ cup pecans, coarsely chopped

6 ounces silken tofu

Juice from 2 lemons

1 small shallot, peeled and chopped

2–3 tablespoons poppy seeds

2 tablespoons sugar

SALAD

1 head romaine lettuce, trimmed, torn, washed, and spun dry

3 cups mesclun greens

Sea salt to taste

Black pepper to taste

2 cups fresh croutons (see page 166)

1. Place the pecans in a small skillet over very low heat. Toast until fragrant and no longer raw tasting, shaking the pan often, approximately 12 minutes. Set aside.

2. Meanwhile, place the tofu, lemon juice, shallot, poppy seeds, and sugar in the work bowl of a food processor fitted with a metal blade. Process until a creamy dressing is formed. Set aside.

3. Combine the romaine lettuce and mesclun in a large salad bowl. Season with sea salt and black pepper. Mix in the croutons. Pour on the dressing and toss thoroughly.

4. Divide the salad among 4 bowls and garnish with pecans.

Romaine Salad with Garlicky Beef and Creamy Avocado Dressing

This is a main-course salad and much more healthful than a traditional fat-laden chef salad. A small amount of meat and a light dressing made creamy with silken tofu make it phytoestrogen rich. Tips: Sliced chicken breast (boneless and skinless) or firm tofu can be substituted for the beef. Also, flank steak is easier to slice if it is very cold.

Preparation: 15 minutes
Cooking: 5 minutes
Yield: 4 main-course servings

SALAD

¼ cup pine nuts

Sea salt to taste

3 teaspoons canola oil, divided

8 ounces flank steak, thinly sliced on the bias

Black pepper to taste

4 cloves garlic, peeled and sliced

2 tablespoons top-quality balsamic vinegar

1 head romaine lettuce, trimmed, torn, washed, and spun dry

1 Belgian endive, trimmed and sliced

1 cucumber, peeled, seeded, and sliced

2 tomatoes, sliced into wedges

DRESSING

6 ounces silken tofu

3 tablespoons orange juice

1 avocado, peeled and pitted

2 tablespoons water

1. Place the pine nuts in a small skillet and sprinkle with sea salt. Toast over very low heat until golden, shaking the pan several times. Set them aside.

2. Heat 2 teaspoons of the oil in a wok over high heat. Sprinkle the flank steak with sea salt and black pepper. Carefully

scatter the meat into the pan and sear it, tossing it 3 or 4 times. Move the meat to one side of the wok.

3. Add the remaining oil to the pan. Place the garlic in the oil and cook for 10 seconds. Stir and garlic together. Add vinegar. Cook the meat for 1 more minute. Transfer the meat to a plate and set aside.

4. Combine the tofu, orange juice, avocado, and water in the work bowl of a food processor fitted with a metal blade. Process until a smooth dressing forms. Season with sea salt and black pepper and set aside.

5. In a large salad bowl combine the romaine lettuce, endive, and cucumber. Pour the dressing onto the greens and toss well.

6. Divide the salad among 4 large plates. Garnish each portion with the flank steak, pine nuts, and tomatoes. Accompany with rustic bread.

Toasting Nuts
Toasting nuts with a sprinkle of sea salt deepens their flavor and removes their raw taste. Nuts can be toasted in a skillet on the stovetop. Place the nuts in a heavy, preferably cast-iron, dry skillet and sprinkle with sea salt. Toast over low heat, shaking the pan often, until golden and fragrant. Large nuts, such as pecans and walnuts, will take about 10 minutes; smaller ones, like pine nuts, about 5 minutes. Pine nuts need to be monitored closely since they can go from being perfectly toasted to burned in an instant.

Romaine and Radicchio Salad with Orange and Almonds

Preparation: 10 minutes
Cooking: 10 minutes
(croutons)
Yield: 4 side-dish servings

This is a refreshing and light summer salad. The orange juice and almonds add flavor but still allow the tastes of the lettuce and radicchio to shine through. This dressing is based upon silken tofu instead of oil, so it is low in fat and calories and rich in phyto-estrogens.

DRESSING
6 ounces silken tofu
Juice from 3 juice oranges
1 small shallot, peeled and chopped
1 teaspoon Dijon mustard

SALAD
¼ cup slivered almonds
1 head romaine lettuce, trimmed, torn, washed, and spun dry
1 medium head radicchio, chopped, washed, and spun dry
Sea salt to taste
Black pepper to taste
2 cups fresh croutons (see page 166)

1. Place the almonds in a small skillet over very low heat. Toast until golden, shaking the pan often, approximately 10 minutes.

2. Meanwhile, place the tofu, orange juice, shallot, and mustard in the work bowl of a food processor fitted with a metal blade. Process until a creamy dressing is formed. Set the dressing aside.

3. Combine the romaine lettuce and radicchio in a large salad bowl. Season with sea salt and black pepper. Mix in the croutons. Pour on the dressing and toss thoroughly.

4. Divide the salad among 4 bowls and garnish with almonds.

"Creamy" Caesar Salad

Impossible but true—a Caesar salad that is low in fat and calories and does not contain raw eggs. This version is based upon silken tofu, so it is low in fat and rich in phytoestrogens. It is so creamy and delicious that no one will know what is missing.

Preparation: 10 minutes
Cooking: 15 minutes
(croutons)
Yield: 4 side-dish servings

CROUTONS
1 12-inch-long loaf of rustic bread
3 cloves garlic, peeled
2 tablespoons, extra-virgin olive oil

DRESSING
Juice from 1½ lemons
1 tablespoon Dijon mustard
4–6 ounces silken tofu
Sea salt to taste
Black pepper to taste

SALAD
1 large head romaine lettuce, trimmed, torn, washed, and
   thoroughly dried
4 ounces grated Parmesan cheese

1. Heat the oven to 400°F. Cut the bread lengthwise in half. Rub the garlic cloves on the inside of the bread. Drizzle the inside of the bread with the 2 tablespoons of the olive oil. Cut the bread into cubes and place on a tray. Bake until crisp, approximately 10 minutes. Set them aside and allow to cool.

2. Meanwhile, combine the lemon juice, mustard, and tofu in the work bowl of a food processor fitted with a metal blade. Process until a smooth dressing forms. Season with sea salt and black pepper.

3. Place the lettuce in a large bowl and pour the dressing on it. Add the croutons to the bowl and toss the salad. Add the Parmesan cheese to the salad and toss once more.

4. Divide the salad among four chilled plates and serve at once.

Chapter 14

Pasta and Pizza

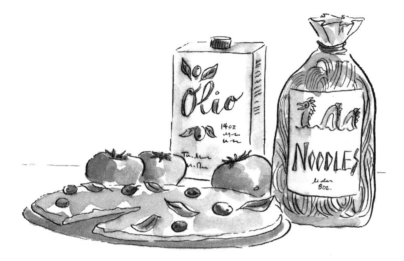

Few foods are as satisfying as a steaming bowl of pasta tossed with a robust sauce, crisp vegetables, and a sharp cheese. Unfortunately, many of the pasta dishes we love are overwhelmed by oil or cream sauces, making them fat-and-calorie–laden affairs. In our recipes the sauces are tofu-based, making them low in fat and calories. When combined with herbs, tomatoes, vegetables, and wonderful cheeses, these light sauces transform an ordinary bowl of noodles into a delectable meal. Besides having a great taste, our pasta dishes are rich in calcium and provide spectacular amounts of phytoestrogens. So why not indulge in Fettuccine with a Tomato "Cream" Sauce, prepared with silken tofu, and fool your friends and family into thinking they are eating the real thing? Or try the Swiss Chard and Mushroom-Filled Shells and see if anyone believes they are eating a tofu-based filling. For those times when you simply want a low-fat pasta meal and are not in the mood for soy, try the Spicy Farfalle with Squid, Tomatoes, and Breadcrumbs.

Pizza is at the top of everybody's favorite-food list. What is more satisfying than a crisp crusted pizza covered with a garlicky tomato sauce and melted mozzarella? Like pasta meals, pizzas, topped with meats and a large amount of cheese, are nutritional nightmares. We have reworked a traditional dough recipe and enhanced it with soy milk and flaxseed to make a wonderful, nutty-tasting, and phytoestrogen-rich pizza crust. Our toppings are tofu-based, giving you a double dose of phytoestrogens in every pie. When you are in the mood to be creative, try the Broccoli-Olive Pesto, Pecan, and Goat Cheese Pizza. For those times when you want a no-fuss pie, simply top your pizza with soy products like soy cheese and soy sausage.

Whether you are in the mood for pasta or pizza, our recipes transform these favorite foods into world-class nutrition and estrogenic feasts.

Grilled Tofu and Vegetables with Chilled Asian Noodles

Marinating: 2 hours
Preparation: 30 minutes
Cooking: 15 minutes
Yield: 4 main-course servings

Tofu is delicious grilled, providing an alternative cooking method for increasing your intake of phytoestrogens. In this recipe it is combined with a variety of vegetables rich in antioxidants, important in fighting cancer. At first glance, with almost 2/3 of a cup of shoyu, this recipe seems high in sodium, but most of it is in the marinade and is not absorbed by the tofu. Tip: This tofu marinade also works well with chicken and beef, especially flank steak. To prevent cross-contamination, chicken and beef should be marinated in separate containers. Also, the noodles can be served chilled or at room temperature.

Tofu and Vegetables

1 pound firm tofu, sliced into 1-inch-thick triangles

½ cup shoyu sauce or tamari

1 tablespoon black-bean garlic sauce or 3 tablespoons oyster sauce

¼ cup water

2 tablespoons rice-wine vinegar

1 tablespoon sugar

3 cloves garlic, peeled and finely chopped

1 2-inch piece gingerroot, peeled and finely chopped

1 medium eggplant, halved and sliced into wedges

1 medium zucchini, halved and sliced into wedges

½ pound asparagus, trimmed

1 large red bell pepper, cored, seeded, and quartered

Noodles

1 cup boiling water

1 ounce dried shiitake mushrooms, stems removed and discarded

Sea salt to taste

12 ounces udon, soba, linguine, or whole-wheat noodles

2 teaspoons canola oil

4 cloves garlic, peeled and thinly sliced

1 1-inch piece gingerroot, peeled and chopped

6 scallions, thinly sliced, white and green parts separated

12 ounces button mushrooms, sliced

3 tablespoons shoyu sauce or tamari

2 tablespoons rice-wine vinegar

2 teaspoons sugar

1 tablespoon sesame oil

1. To marinate the tofu, first place it in a shallow bowl. In another bowl combine the shoyu, black-bean or oyster sauce, water, vinegar, sugar, garlic, and gingerroot and whisk well. Pour ½ of the marinade over the tofu; reserve the other half for the vegetables. Marinate 2 hours, turning occasionally.

2. To prepare the noodles, pour the boiling water on the shiitake

mushrooms. Allow them to macerate for 20 minutes. Drain them and reserve their soaking water. Slice the caps and set aside.

3. Meanwhile, bring a large pot of water to a boil. Add sea salt to the water, followed by the noodles.

4. Heat the canola oil in a wok over low heat. Add the garlic and gingerroot and cook them until soft and fragrant, stirring occasionally.

5. Raise the heat to high and add the white parts of the scallions and the button mushrooms to the wok. Cook until the mushrooms are soft and all of their liquid has evaporated. Add shoyu, rice wine vinegar, sugar, shiitake mushrooms, and their soaking water. Bring sauce to a boil, reduce heat, and simmer for 3 minutes. Stir in the green parts of the scallions.

6. Drain the noodles and transfer them to the wok. Cook the noodles and sauce together for 2 minutes over low heat, stirring occasionally. Add the sesame oil to the noodles. Transfer them to a large bowl and allow them to cool.

7. To prepare the vegetables, pour the remaining marinade on them. Light a hardwood fire. Allow the coals to ash over. Grill the vegetables and tofu until they are tender, approximately 15 minutes. Slice each square of tofu into three strips and cut the vegetables into 3-inch pieces.

8. Divide the pasta evenly among four plates and garnish with the tofu and vegetables.

Shoyu
Many commercially produced soy sauces are not fermented and are derived from hydrolyzed vegetable protein, corn syrup, caramel color, salt, and MSG. Shoyu, Japanese in origin, is a naturally fermented soy sauce containing only soybeans, wheat, and salt. It is the seasoning we prefer to use. If you cannot find it, tamari is a good substitute. Tamari, the Chinese version of shoyu, sometimes is made without wheat.

Spaghetti with a Tomato-Tofu Sauce

Everyone has a "spaghetti and sauce" recipe in their repertoire. It is a great meal because it is quick and nutritious, and the ingredients probably are on hand. Here is our version, tailored to meet the phytoestrogenic needs of menopause. Tips: *You can substitute one tablespoon of dried basil and 1 teaspoon of dried oregano for the fresh herbs. Add them to the onion after it has been softened and cook them for 2 minutes before you proceed with the recipe. Also, if desired, you can add 10 finely chopped green or black olives to the sauce while it simmers.*

Preparation: 10 minutes
Cooking: 30 minutes
Yield: 4 main-course servings

2 tablespoons olive oil, divided
6 cloves garlic, peeled and sliced
1 yellow onion, peeled and diced
Sea salt to taste
1 28-ounce can whole tomatoes, chopped
1 pound firm tofu, cut into small cubes
4 tablespoons top-quality red-wine vinegar
Black pepper to taste
½ cup fresh basil, snipped
2 tablespoons fresh oregano, chopped
1 pound spaghetti
4 tablespoons grated Parmesan cheese

1. Bring a large pot of water to a boil. Heat 1 tablespoon of the olive oil in a Dutch oven over low heat. Add the garlic and cook until soft and fragrant. Add the onion to the Dutch oven and sprinkle with sea salt. Cook the onion until soft, stirring occasionally.

2. Raise the heat to high and add the tomatoes to the Dutch oven. Bring the sauce to a boil, reduce the heat, and simmer for 15 minutes, stirring occasionally.

3. Meanwhile, heat the remaining olive oil in a well-seasoned wok over high heat. When the oil is hot, place the tofu in the wok. Cook until golden, stirring several times. Add the

vinegar to the wok and cook the tofu for 30 seconds more. Season with sea salt and black pepper and add it to the sauce. Cook the sauce for 5 minutes more. Remove the sauce from the heat and stir in the basil and oregano. Season the sauce with sea salt and black pepper.

4. Add sea salt to the boiling water, followed by the pasta. Cook the pasta until tender. Drain and divide among 4 plates. Spoon the sauce and tofu onto each plate and garnish with Parmesan cheese.

Canned Tomatoes
Several recipes in this book call for canned tomatoes. Top-quality canned tomatoes are a staple in our kitchen. Unfortunately, significant differences in quality are found in the large selection of tomatoes available. The best are those from the San Marzano region in Italy. San Marzano plum tomatoes are grown specifically for cooking, but beware: Some producers claim their tomatoes are "San Marzano Type" or "San Marzano Quality." If San Marzano tomatoes are not available, we suggest trying several brands to find a brand you enjoy. Search for a can that contains deep-red tomatoes that are neither too soft nor too firm, with little or no added salt and a clean tomato flavor.

Linguine with Littleneck Clams, Spicy Sausage, and Tomatoes

Contrary to popular belief, most shellfish are not high in choles-terol. Clams are much lower in cholesterol than meat, poultry, eggs, and cheese. In this recipe we have substituted chicken or turkey sausage for the traditional pork sausage to keep the satu-rated-fat content lower and have added phytoestrogen-rich silken tofu to enhance the texture of the sauce. So you can try this dish—one not usually thought of as heart-healthy—with a light heart. Tips: The sauce, without the clams, tofu, and basil can be pre-pared one day in advance, covered, and refrigerated. Also, when seasoning the sauce with sea salt, keep in mind that the liquid from the clams is salty.

Preparation: 15 minutes
Cooking: 45 minutes
Yield: 6 main-course servings

2 tablespoons olive oil, divided

12 ounces chicken or turkey andouille sausage, sliced

5 cloves garlic, peeled and sliced

1 onion, diced

½ Scotch bonnet pepper, seeded and finely chopped

⅔ cup dry white wine

1 28-ounce can whole tomatoes, chopped

Sea salt to taste

1 pound linguine

36 littleneck clams, scrubbed and rinsed

½ cup fresh basil, snipped

8 ounces silken tofu, pureed

Black pepper to taste

1. Heat 1 tablespoon of the olive oil in a large Dutch oven over high heat. Carefully place the sausage in the pot and sear it, stirring 3 or 4 times. Remove from the pot and set aside.

2. Heat the remaining olive oil in the pot over low heat. Add the garlic and cook it until soft and fragrant. Add the

onion and Scotch bonnet pepper and cook until the onion is soft, stirring often.

3. Raise the heat to high and add the wine to the pot and simmer for 3 minutes. Return the sausage and any accumulated juices to the pot. Add the tomatoes and bring to a boil. Reduce the heat and simmer the sauce for 20 minutes, stirring occasionally.

4. While the sauce is simmering, bring a large pot of water to a boil. Add sea salt to the water, followed by the pasta.

5. Raise the heat to high under the sauce and bring to a boil. Carefully place the clams in the sauce and cover the pot.

6. As the clams open, remove them from the sauce. Reduce the heat and add the basil and tofu to the sauce. Season with sea salt and black pepper.

7. Drain the pasta and add it to the sauce. Cook the pasta and sauce together for 2 minutes, stirring often.

8. Divide the pasta and sauce among six shallow bowls. Garnish with clams and serve immediately.

Searing

Searing is browning the surface of meat, fish, poultry, or tofu over high heat in a small amount of oil. It works best in an uncrowded pan and with food that has been thoroughly dried. The particles that remain on the bottom of the pan after you remove the seared food are ideal for making a sauce. Deglaze the pan with water, wine, or stock and scrape the particles with a spoon to dissolve them.

Farfalle with Caramelized Butternut Squash and Tofu, Mustard Greens, and Blue Cheese

Roasted vegetables are a real treat. The process brings out the natural sweetness of squash. Here the tofu is added to the roasting vegetables, which makes it crisp and sweet, another unique and delicious way to enjoy this phytoestrogen-rich food. Mustard greens, along with tofu and blue cheese, make this a calcium-rich meal. Tips: *The majority of the preparation is allocated to the roasting of the squash and tofu. To save time, roast them a day in advance. The following day heat them in the oven while the pasta is cooking. Also, to clean the roasting pan, fill it with hot water and place it in the oven. Allow the pan to sit for a day or two. The hardened pieces of brown sugar will dissolve, and the pan will be easier to clean.*

Preparation: 45 minutes
Cooking: 15 minutes
Yield: 6 main-course servings

1 large butternut squash, peeled, seeded, and sliced into ½-inch cubes

1 pound firm tofu, cut into 1-inch cubes

3 tablespoons olive oil, divided

⅓ cup dark brown sugar

Sea salt to taste

Black pepper to taste

1 pound farfalle

2 cloves garlic, peeled and thinly sliced

1½ pounds mustard greens, trimmed, chopped, washed, and drained

½ cup pasta-cooking water

6 ounces Blue Castello, room temperature

1. Heat the oven to 400°F.
2. Place the squash and tofu in a large bowl. Drizzle with

two tablespoons of the olive oil and sprinkle with brown sugar, sea salt, and black pepper. Transfer to a heavy baking tray. Roast the ingredients until very soft and caramelized, stirring several times, approximately 40 minutes. Remove the tray from the oven and loosen the ingredients with a spatula. Set aside.

3. While the squash and tofu are roasting, bring a large pot of water to a boil. Add sea salt to the water, followed by the pasta.

4. Heat the remaining tablespoon of olive oil in a Dutch oven over low heat. Add the garlic to the oil and cook until soft and fragrant.

5. Raise the heat to high and add the mustard greens to the Dutch oven. Sprinkle with sea salt and cover. Steam the greens for 3 minutes. Add the pasta-cooking water to the greens.

6. Drain the pasta and add it to the greens. Reduce the heat to low and cook the pasta and greens together for 2 minutes, stirring often. Season with sea salt and black pepper.

7. Divide the pasta, squash, and tofu among 6 shallow bowls. Garnish with blue cheese.

Linguine with Mushrooms and Parsley

Preparation: 25 minutes
Cooking: 15 minutes
Yield: 4 main-course servings

After tasting this creamy pasta dish, you may think the title of the recipe should have included cream, but cream is not an ingredient. Silken tofu has been used to provide phytoestrogens and a creamy texture, also making this recipe very heart healthy. Tip: *An efficient method to remove the stems from dried shiitake mushrooms is to snap them off while they are still dry.*

¼ ounce dried shiitake mushrooms, stems removed and
    discarded
¼ ounce dried porcini mushrooms
1 cup boiling water

1 tablespoon olive oil

6 cloves garlic, peeled and sliced

8 ounces white button mushrooms, sliced

8 ounces crimini mushrooms, sliced

Sea salt to taste

12 ounces linguine

½ cup dry white wine

Mushroom-soaking water

½ cup flat-leaf parsley, chopped

4 ounces silken tofu, pureed

Black pepper to taste

4 tablespoons grated Romano cheese

1. Place the shiitake and porcini mushrooms in a bowl. Pour the boiling water on them and cover the bowl tightly. Allow them to soften for 15 minutes. Drain them and reserve their soaking water. Chop the mushrooms and set aside.

2. Bring a large pot of water to a boil. While the mushrooms are softening, heat the olive oil in a Dutch oven over high heat. Add the garlic to the Dutch oven and cook for 30 seconds, stirring constantly. Add the white and crimini mushrooms and sprinkle with sea salt. Cook the mushrooms until soft and all of their liquid has evaporated, approximately 5 minutes.

3. Add sea salt to the boiling water, followed by the pasta. Add the wine to the mushrooms in the Dutch oven and simmer for 3 minutes. Add the mushroom-soaking water and dried mushrooms. Stir in the parsley and cook the sauce for 1 minute.

4. Stir the pureed tofu into the sauce. Drain the pasta and add to the sauce.

5. Reduce the heat to low and cook the pasta and sauce together for 2 minutes. Season with sea salt and black pepper.

6. Divide the pasta among 4 plates and garnish with Romano cheese.

Cooking and Saucing Pasta

Several important techniques will help you successfully cook and sauce a pasta meal. First, start with plenty of rapidly boiling water—about 4 quarts for 1 pound of pasta. A small amount of salt added to the water before the pasta is added will give the pasta a well-rounded flavor. Next, cover the pot immediately after you have added the noodles and uncover it once the water has returned to a boil. When testing pasta for doneness, taste a piece and keep in mind whether it is going to require additional cooking (e.g., manicotti, lasagna, and stuffed shells will be baked in the oven). Fresh pasta cooks very quickly, and it is usually done when the water returns to a boil or when the noodles float to the surface.

Pasta needs to be rinsed only if it is being used in a cold salad. When preparing a cold pasta salad that contains an acid, such as vinegar or lemon juice, remember that the acid will continue to cook the noodles. Also, coating cooked pasta with oil will cause a poor adhesion between the sauce and noodles. Last, when saucing pasta with a thick tomato-based sauce, it is fine to ladle the sauce on top of the cooked noodles. When you have a sauce that consists of oil, butter, and cream or any combination of the three, stir the cooked noodles directly into the sauce and heat them together for two minutes over low heat. That will ensure a perfect marriage between the sauce and noodles.

Swiss Chard and Mushroom–Filled Shells

Preparation: 40 minutes
Cooking: 20 minutes
Yield: 6 main-course
servings

We have substituted pureed tofu for ricotta and soy mozzarella for dairy mozzarella and have added Swiss chard to the filling of a traditional stuffed-shell recipe. The filling retains its creamy tex-

ture and flavor, and our version is a great source of phytoestrogens and calcium. Tip: *Both parts of this recipe, sauce and filling, can be prepared a day in advance.*

SAUCE

1 tablespoon olive oil

5 cloves garlic, peeled and sliced

1 onion, peeled and diced

Sea salt to taste

½ cup dry red wine

1 28-ounce can whole tomatoes, chopped

½ cup flat-leaf parsley, chopped

Black pepper to taste

SHELLS AND FILLING

Sea salt to taste

12 ounces large (stuffing) shells

1 tablespoon olive oil

4 cloves garlic, peeled and sliced

1 onion, peeled and diced

1 pound white mushrooms, sliced

1 pound green Swiss chard, trimmed, chopped, washed, and drained

Black pepper to taste

2 pounds silken tofu

⅓ cup grated Romano cheese

1 egg yolk

6 ounces soy mozzarella cheese, grated or sliced

1. To prepare the sauce, heat the olive oil in a Dutch oven over low heat. Add the garlic to the oil and cook until soft and fragrant.

2. Add the onion to the pot and sprinkle with sea salt. Cook the onion until soft, stirring occasionally. Raise the heat to high and add the wine. Simmer for 2 minutes.

3. Add the tomatoes to the pot and bring to a boil. Reduce the heat and simmer for 20 minutes, stirring occasionally. Add

the parsley to the sauce. Season with sea salt and black pepper. Set aside.

4. While the sauce is simmering, bring a large pot of water to a boil. Add sea salt to the water, followed by the shells. Cook the shells until tender but still a bit firm. They will soften more when they are baked. Rinse the shells under cold water and set aside.

5. While the sauce is simmering and the shells are cooking, prepare the filling. Heat the olive oil in a wok over low heat. Add the garlic to the oil and cook it until soft and fragrant. Add the onion to the wok and cook until it is soft, stirring occasionally.

6. Raise the heat to high and add the mushrooms to the wok. Sprinkle the mushrooms with sea salt and cook until soft, approximately 5 minutes. Heat the oven to 400°F.

7. Add the chard to the wok. Reduce the heat slightly and cover the pan. Steam the chard until tender, stirring often. If necessary, add water to the chard to prevent it from sticking. Remove the cover from the wok and cook the chard for 2 minutes longer, stirring often. Season with sea salt and black pepper. Transfer the ingredients to a large plate and place in the refrigerator to cool.

8. Combine the tofu, Romano cheese, and yolk in the work bowl of a food processor fitted with a metal blade. Process until smooth. Transfer to a large bowl. Press any moisture out of the mushroom-chard mixture. Stir the vegetables into the tofu.

9. Fill the shells with the vegetable-tofu mixture and transfer to a large oven-proof casserole. Top the shells with the sauce and mozzarella cheese. Bake the shells until the cheese melts and they are heated through, approximately 20 minutes.

10. Divide the shells among 6 plates. Accompany with a green salad and rustic bread.

Swiss Chard

Earthy tasting leaves and sweet stems make Swiss chard a staple in our kitchen. Calcium-rich chard is also an excellent source of iron, folate, potassium, and vitamin A.

The two varieties of chard are white and red; they are interchangeable in recipes, but keep in mind that red chard will bleed when cooked. Swiss chard can be added to soups, tossed with pasta, or used as a topping for pizza. It is at its best, though, when cooked in olive oil and garlic and served as a side dish. A squeeze of lemon and a sprinkling of toasted pine nuts are wonderful additions.

To prepare chard for cooking, trim, chop, and wash it well. Since the stems take longer to soften than the leaves, it is helpful but not critical to separate them. If you do not separate them, allow a few extra minutes of cooking for the stems to soften. You can treat chard like spinach and cook it only until the stems are soft and the leaves wilt. However, unlike spinach, chard benefits from a long cooking time. If you are fortunate enough to find or grow baby chard, it is wonderful in a green salad.

Mushroom and Fennel Ragu

A ragu is traditionally a meat-based, slow-cooked tomato sauce served with polenta or pasta. This version is prepared with tempeh in place of the meat. It has a surprisingly "meaty" taste, as the tempeh takes on the flavors from the sauce. Tips: *Firm tofu can be substituted for the tempeh. The sauce can be prepared 2 days in advance and refrigerated. That not only is convenient but also improves the flavor.*

Preparation: 15 minutes
Cooking: 1 hour
Yield: 4 main-course servings

1 ounce dried porcini mushrooms

1 cup boiling water

1 tablespoon olive oil

4 cloves garlic, peeled and sliced

1 onion, peeled and diced

1 bulb fennel, trimmed and diced

Sea salt to taste

½ pound portobello mushrooms, stems removed, caps wiped
   clean and sliced

12 ounces tempeh, cut into small cubes

1 cup dry red wine

Mushroom-soaking liquid

1 28-ounce can whole tomatoes, chopped

½ cup flat-leaf parsley, chopped

Black pepper to taste

1. Place the porcini mushrooms in a bowl and pour the boiling water on them. Allow them to macerate for 20 minutes. Drain them and reserve their soaking water.

2. Meanwhile, heat the olive oil in a Dutch oven over low heat. Add the garlic to the pot and cook until soft and fragrant. Add the onion to the pot and cook until soft, stirring occasionally.

3. Add the fennel to the pot and a pinch of sea salt. Cover the pot and steam the fennel until soft, stirring occasionally. Add the portobellos to the pot and cook until soft. Stir in the tempeh and porcini mushrooms.

4. Raise the heat to high and add the wine and mushroom-soaking liquid. Simmer the mixture for 3 minutes.

5. Add the tomatoes and bring the sauce to a boil. Reduce the heat, cover the pot, and simmer for 45 minutes, stirring occasionally. Remove the cover from the pot and simmer for 15 minutes longer.

6. Stir in the parsley and season the ragu with sea salt and black pepper. Divide the ragu among 4 shallow bowls. Accompany with Polenta (see page 272).

Fettuccine with a Tomato "Cream" Sauce

Silken tofu makes a great substitute for cream in a pasta sauce. This smooth sauce is tomato-based, making it rich in the antioxidant vitamin C. Tip: *The sauce can be prepared a day in advance. The following day heat the sauce slowly, and just before draining the pasta, add a cup of its cooking water to the sauce.*

Preparation: 10 minutes
Cooking: 20 minutes
Yield: 6 side-dish servings

1 tablespoon olive oil
4 cloves garlic, peeled and sliced
1 onion, peeled and diced
Sea salt to taste
1 28-ounce can whole tomatoes, drained and chopped
2 tablespoons fresh oregano, chopped
8 ounces silken tofu
Black pepper to taste
1 pound fettuccine
6 tablespoons grated Romano cheese

1. Heat the olive oil in a Dutch oven over low heat. Add the garlic cloves to the pot and cook them until they are soft and fragrant. Add the onion to the pot, sprinkle it with sea salt, and cook it until it is soft.

2. Raise the heat to high, add the tomatoes to the pot, and bring the sauce to a boil. Reduce the heat and simmer for 20 minutes, stirring occasionally. While the sauce is simmering, bring a large pot of water to a boil.

3. Transfer the sauce to the work bowl of a food processor fitted with a metal blade. Add the oregano to the sauce and puree the sauce. Add the tofu to the work bowl and process the sauce until smooth. Season with sea salt and black pepper. Return the sauce to the pot.

4. Add sea salt to the boiling water, followed by the pasta.

Cook the pasta until tender. Drain the pasta, reserving 1 cup of its cooking water.

5. Add the cooking water to the sauce, followed by the pasta, and stir the ingredients thoroughly. Divide the pasta among 6 bowls and garnish with Romano cheese.

Spicy Farfalle with Squid, Tomatoes, and Breadcrumbs

Preparation: 15 minutes
Cooking: 35 minutes
Yield: 6 main-course servings

Squid are a bit higher in cholesterol than other fish but still low in saturated fat. This hearty and spicy dish is quite low in calories. Tips: *The best pot to use is a cast-iron Dutch oven. Both the sauce and the breadcrumbs can be prepared a day in advance and refrigerated. Also, to reduce the spiciness of the Scotch bonnet pepper, remove its seeds and ribs. To be safe, wash and dry your hands and cutting board thoroughly after working with the pepper. Some cooks suggest wearing plastic gloves when you are working with such fiery chilies.*

2 cups fresh breadcrumbs
⅓ cup flat-leaf parsley
8 cloves garlic, peeled, sliced, and divided
Sea salt to taste
Black pepper to taste
2 tablespoons olive oil, divided
½–1 Scotch bonnet chili, seeded and finely chopped
¾ cup white wine
1 28-ounce can whole tomatoes, drained and chopped
1 pound farfalle
1 pound squid bodies and tentacles, sliced
½ cup cilantro, chopped

1. Combine the breadcrumbs, parsley, 2 cloves of garlic, sea salt, black pepper, and 1 tablespoon of olive oil in the work

bowl of a food processor that is fitted with a metal blade. Process the ingredients until well combined.

2. Heat the broiler. Bring a large pot of water to a boil on the stove. Heat the remaining tablespoon of olive oil in a Dutch oven over low heat. Add the remaining 6 cloves of garlic and cook them until they are soft and fragrant, stirring constantly. Add the chili to the pot and cook the ingredients for two minutes, stirring often.

3. Raise the heat to high and pour in the wine. Simmer for two minutes. Stir in the tomatoes and bring the sauce to a boil. Reduce the heat and simmer for 10 minutes.

4. While the sauce is simmering, add sea salt to the boiling water, followed by the pasta.

5. Raise the heat to high under the sauce and stir in the squid and cilantro. Cook the squid until they are bright white, approximately 2 minutes. Drain the pasta and add it to the sauce in the Dutch oven.

6. Remove the pot from the heat and season the pasta with sea salt and black pepper. Scatter the seasoned breadcrumbs on the pasta and press them slightly. Place the pot under the broiler and cook the pasta until the breadcrumbs are golden, approximately 5 minutes.

7. Divide the pasta among 6 plates and accompany with rustic bread.

Whole-Wheat Penne with Turkey Andouille Sausage and Swiss Chard

Substituting whole-wheat pasta for white pasta is an excellent way to boost the fiber content of your diet. In order to keep this dish low in fat, we have replaced the more traditional pork sausage with turkey sausage. Swiss chard is an excellent source of antioxidants, important in preventing cancer. Tip: *If you can't get*

Preparation: 10 minutes
Cooking: 20 minutes
Yield: 4 main-course servings

turkey andouille sausage, you can use a sweet or hot Italian turkey sausage.

1 tablespoon plus 1 teaspoon olive oil, divided
8 ounces turkey andouille sausage, sliced into ½-inch-thick disks
Sea salt to taste
1 pound whole-wheat penne
5 cloves garlic, peeled and sliced
1 pound green Swiss chard, trimmed, washed, and drained, stems sliced into matchsticks and leaves chopped
1½ cups low-sodium chicken broth
Black pepper to taste
4 tablespoons grated Parmesan cheese

1. Bring a large pot of water to a boil. Heat 1 tablespoon of the oil in a wok over high heat. When the oil is hot, add the sausage. Sear the sausage on both sides, turning it 2 or 3 times. Remove and set aside.

2. Add sea salt to the water, followed by the pasta. Heat the remaining oil in the wok over low heat. Add the garlic to the wok and cook it until soft and fragrant, stirring occasionally.

3. Raise the heat to high and add the chard to the wok. Cook for 2 minutes, stirring often. Add the chicken broth. Return the sausage to the wok and cover the pan.

4. Cook the ingredients until the chard is tender, stirring occasionally. Drain the pasta and add to the wok. Reduce the heat and cook the pasta and sauce together for 2 minutes. Season with sea salt and black pepper.

5. Divide the pasta among 4 shallow bowls and garnish with Parmesan cheese.

Canned Chicken Broth

It is difficult to be so organized in our cooking that we always have a supply of homemade chicken broth at the ready to use in our favorite recipes. The alternative is using canned chicken broth. Nevertheless, finding a flavorful and healthful canned broth is challenging. As with canned tomatoes, the quality of canned broths varies significantly. The most obvious downfall of a canned broth is too much sodium. Many taste like salted water. Look for a canned broth low in sodium (60 milligrams or less for an 8-ounce serving), with only spices and dehydrated vegetables as the added ingredients.

Farfalle with Tofu, Broccoli Rabe, Dried Tomatoes, Corn, and Goat Cheese

At first glance you may not realize that this dish is rich in calcium. Both broccoli rabe and corn are good vegetarian sources of calcium, while goat cheese is an excellent dairy source. This pasta dish is an example of contrasting tastes making a delicious whole. The pungent broccoli rabe and sweet tomatoes and tofu are a perfect complement for the mellow goat cheese. Tips: *If you don't care for the sharp taste of broccoli rabe, a milder-flavored green, such as Swiss chard, is a fine substitute. Also, when fresh corn is in season, be sure to use it in this recipe.*

Preparation: 15 minutes
Cooking: 15 minutes
Yield: 4 main-course servings

1 cup dried tomatoes
1 cup boiling water
Sea salt to taste
1 pound farfalle
2 tablespoons olive oil, divided
1 pound firm tofu, cut into small cubes
3 tablespoons top-quality balsamic vinegar
6 cloves garlic, peeled and sliced
1½ pounds broccoli rabe, trimmed and rinsed
Tomato-soaking water
1½ cups frozen corn kernels or kernels from 3 ears of fresh
    corn (see box on page 197)
Black pepper to taste
4 ounces goat cheese at room temperature

1. Place the dried tomatoes in a bowl and pour the boiling water on them. Allow them to macerate for 10 minutes or until they are soft. Drain them and reserve their soaking water. Coarsely chop the tomatoes and set aside.

2. Meanwhile, bring a large pot of water to a boil. Add sea salt to the water, followed by the pasta.

3. While the pasta is cooking, heat 1 tablespoon of the olive oil in a wok over high heat. When the oil is hot, add the tofu. Cook the tofu until golden, stirring several times. Add the vinegar to the wok and cook the tofu for 30 more seconds. Transfer the tofu to a plate and set aside.

4. Heat the remaining tablespoon of oil in the wok over low heat. Add the garlic to the pan and cook until soft and fragrant, stirring occasionally.

5. Raise the heat to high and add the broccoli rabe to the pot and a dash of sea salt. Stir the broccoli rabe, cover the pot, and steam for 2 minutes. Add the reserved tomato-soaking water to the pot and cook the broccoli rabe until tender.

6. Add the corn and the dried tomatoes to the pot. Drain the pasta and add to the vegetables. Reduce the heat to low and cook the pasta and vegetables together for 2 minutes. Season with sea salt and black pepper.

7. Divide the pasta among 4 shallow bowls and garnish with the tofu and goat cheese.

Removing the Kernels from an Ear of Corn
To cut the kernels of a corn cob, stand an ear upright with the stem end resting securely on a cutting board. With a sharp, broad-bladed knife, cut off the top half of the kernels as you move your knife down the ear. Next, with the back side of the knife, repeat the procedure with more pressure to remove the bottom portion of the kernels and the wonderful corn juices.

Whole-Wheat Penne with Asparagus, Chicken, and Lemon

This light and delicious pasta meal is rich in fiber from the whole-wheat pasta and asparagus. Chicken with the skin removed is low in saturated fat, making it heart healthy. Tip: *When selecting asparagus, keep in mind that those with thin stems will be most tender.*

Preparation: 10 minutes
Cooking: 15 minutes
Yield: 4 main-course servings

1 cup water
Sea salt to taste
1 pound asparagus, trimmed, each stalk sliced into 3 diagonal pieces
¼ cup slivered almonds
12 ounces whole-wheat penne
4 teaspoons olive oil, divided
¾ pound boneless, skinless chicken breast, thinly sliced
Juice from 2 lemons
⅓ cup fresh basil, snipped
3 large shallots, peeled and chopped
Reserved asparagus-steaming water
Black pepper to taste
4 tablespoons grated Parmesan cheese

1. Bring a large pot of water to a boil.

2. Place 1 cup of water in a Dutch oven and bring to a boil. Add dash of sea salt. Place the asparagus in the water and cover the pot. Steam the asparagus until tender, approximately 4 minutes. Drain it, reserving the steaming water. Cool the asparagus under running water and set aside.

3. While the asparagus is steaming, place the almonds in a small skillet and sprinkle with sea salt. Toast the almonds over low heat until golden, shaking the skillet often. Set the almonds aside.

4. Add sea salt to the boiling water, followed by the pasta.

5. Heat 2 teaspoons of the olive oil in a wok over high heat. When the oil is hot, add the chicken to the wok. Sear the chicken, stirring it 3 or 4 times. Add the lemon juice and cook the chicken for another minute. Remove the wok from the heat and add the basil to the chicken. Transfer the chicken to a plate.

6. Heat the remaining 2 teaspoons of olive oil in the skillet over low heat. Add the shallots to the skillet and cook until they are soft, stirring occasionally.

7. Raise the heat to high and add the reserved asparagus steaming water to the skillet. Bring the liquid to a boil and add the asparagus.

8. Drain the pasta and add it to the wok. Return the chicken to the wok. Add the asparagus mixture to the wok. Cook the pasta and asparagus-shallot sauce together for 2 minutes. Season with sea salt and black pepper.

9. Divide the pasta among 4 plates and garnish with Parmesan cheese.

Penne with Eggplant, Tomato, and Tofu Sauce

If you enjoy eggplant as much as we do, you will love this quick eggplant sauce. Red-wine-vinegar–flavored tofu provides flavor, texture, and, of course, phytoestrogens. Tips: *A more efficient method would be to eliminate step 4 and cook the eggplant with the onions and garlic in step 1; we believe the eggplant loses its character if it is cooked in that manner. When the eggplant is cooked separately in a hot pan, it retains its texture and takes on a smoky flavor. Also, leftovers are wonderful in a baguette with melted mozzarella.*

Preparation: 10 minutes
Cooking: 35 minutes
Yield: 4 main-course servings

2 teaspoons plus 2 tablespoons olive oil, divided
6 cloves garlic, peeled and sliced
1 yellow onion, peeled and diced
1 28-ounce can whole tomatoes, chopped
Sea salt to taste
1 pound penne
1 pound firm tofu, sliced into small cubes
4 tablespoons top-quality red-wine vinegar
2½ pounds Japanese or Italian eggplant, cubed
½ cup fresh basil, snipped
Black pepper to taste
4 tablespoons grated Parmesan cheese

1. Heat 2 teaspoons of the olive oil in a Dutch oven over low heat. Add the garlic and cook until soft and fragrant. Add the onion to the pot and cook until soft.

2. Raise the heat to high and add the tomatoes to the pot. Bring the sauce to a boil, reduce the heat, and simmer for 20 minutes. Bring a large pot of water to a boil. Add sea salt to the water, followed by the penne.

3. Meanwhile, heat 1 tablespoon of the olive oil in a well-seasoned wok over high heat. When the oil is hot, add the tofu to the pan. Cook until golden, stirring 3 or 4 times. Sprinkle the tofu with sea salt and add the vinegar to the pan. Cook for 15 more seconds. Transfer the tofu to a plate and set aside.

4. Heat the remaining tablespoon of oil in the wok over high heat. When the oil is hot, add the eggplant to the pan, and sprinkle with sea salt. Cook the eggplant until golden and smoky, stirring several times. Stir the eggplant into the tomato sauce and cook for 10 more minutes.

5. Stir the basil into the sauce and season with sea salt and black pepper. Drain the pasta and divide it among 4 plates. Ladle sauce onto each portion and garnish with tofu and Parmesan cheese.

Linguine with Lemon, Pepper, Tofu, and Chard

Preparation: 10 minutes
Cooking: 15 minutes
Yield: 4 main-course servings

Lemon, black pepper, and fresh herbs are a wonderful combination. These ingredients often are paired with chicken or shrimp; we have discovered that they also work well with tofu. This quick pasta dish has phytoestrogens and plenty of calcium from Parmesan cheese, one of the best cheese sources of calcium. Tip: Feel free to vary the herb. Thyme, tarragon, and oregano, all in smaller quantities (about 2 tablespoons), work well. Also, spinach can be substituted for the chard.

Sea salt to taste
1 pound linguine
2 tablespoons plus 2 teaspoons olive oil, divided

1 pound firm tofu, sliced into small cubes

Black pepper to taste

Juice from 1½ lemons

½ cup fresh basil, snipped

4 shallots, peeled and chopped (approximately 1/4 cup)

4 cloves garlic, peeled and sliced

1½ pounds chard, trimmed, washed and drained, stems
   julienned and leaves chopped

1 cup pasta-cooking water

4 tablespoons grated Parmesan cheese

1. Bring a large pot of water to a boil. Add sea salt to the water, followed by the pasta.

2. While the pasta is cooking, heat 1 tablespoon of the olive oil in a well-seasoned wok over high heat. When the oil is hot, add the tofu to the wok. Cook the tofu until golden, stirring several times. Sprinkle with sea salt and black pepper. Add the lemon juice and basil. Cook for 30 more seconds. Remove the tofu from the wok and set aside.

3. Reduce the heat to low under the wok. Add 2 more teaspoons of olive oil to the wok. Add the shallots and cook until they are soft. Return the tofu to the wok and combine it with the shallots. Remove the tofu and set aside.

4. Heat the remaining tablespoon of oil in the wok over high heat. Add the garlic to the pan and cook for 30 seconds, stirring constantly. Add the chard to the wok and cover the pan. Steam the chard for 5 minutes, stirring often. Add the pasta-cooking water to the chard and cook the chard until it is tender.

5. Drain the pasta and place it in the wok. Reduce the heat to low under the wok and cook the pasta and chard together for 1 minute.

6. Divide the pasta among 4 bowls. Garnish with Parmesan cheese and the tofu.

Linguine with Tofu, Flank Steak, Bok Choy, and Asparagus

Preparation: 15 minutes
Cooking: 10 minutes
Yield: 4 main-course servings

Like much of Asian cookery, the beef in this recipe is used more as a garnish than as the main component of the dish; the tofu absorbs the wonderful flavors and adds texture. This manner of cooking allows you to keep beef as a part of your diet, without adding excess fat and cholesterol. Bok choy and asparagus are both rich sources of antioxidants and folic acid, a B-vitamin important in heart disease prevention.

4 tablespoons oyster sauce

4 tablespoons shoyu sauce or tamari

4 tablespoons orange juice

1½ cups low-sodium chicken broth

1 teaspoon sugar

2 teaspoons sesame oil

1½ cups water

Sea salt to taste

1 pound asparagus, trimmed, each stalk sliced into 3
   diagonal pieces

1 pound linguine

2 tablespoons canola oil, divided

8 ounces flank steak, thinly sliced on the bias

8 ounces firm tofu, cut into small cubes

4 cloves garlic, peeled and sliced

1 1-inch piece gingerroot peeled and minced

8 ounces white mushrooms, sliced

1 red bell pepper, cored and sliced

½ pound bok choy, trimmed, stems sliced diagonally into
   ¾-inch-thick pieces and leaves coarsely chopped

4 tablespoons Spicy Soy Nuts (see page 274), optional

1. In a bowl whisk together the oyster sauce, shoyu, orange juice, chicken broth, sugar, and sesame oil. Set aside.

2. Bring the 1½ cups of water to a boil. Add a dash of sea salt. Place the asparagus in the water and cover the pot. Steam the asparagus until bright green and tender. Drain and cool under running water. Set aside.

3. Bring a large pot of water to a boil. Add sea salt, followed by the pasta.

4. Heat 1 tablespoon of the canola oil in a wok over high heat. When the oil is hot, scatter the flank steak and tofu around the pan. Cook the ingredients until golden, turning them 2 or 3 times. Whisk the sauce and add 1/2 cup of it to the wok. Cook for 30 seconds more. Transfer to a plate and set aside.

5. Heat the remaining tablespoon of canola oil in the wok and add the garlic and gingerroot to the pan. Cook for 30 seconds. Add the mushrooms, bell pepper, and bok choy to the pan. Cook the vegetables for 4 minutes, stirring often.

6. Add the remaining sauce to the wok. Bring the sauce to a boil, reduce the heat, and simmer for 2 minutes. Add the flank steak, tofu, and asparagus to the sauce.

7. Drain the pasta and add it to the wok. Cook the pasta and sauce together for 2 minutes. Divide the pasta among 4 plates and, if desired, garnish with Spicy Soy Nuts (see page 274).

Pappardelle with Pork, Escarole, and Blue Cheese

This recipe, Hope's favorite, is arguably the most delicious in this book. A pig's diet has undergone dramatic changes over the years, making pork a relatively low-fat meat as long as a lean cut, such as the loin in this recipe, is used. Escarole is a rich source of antioxidants; it adds an earthy and slightly sharp flavor to the dish. Tip: We tested this recipe with fresh pappardelle (wide noodles). If it is not available, fresh or dried fettuccine can be substituted.

Preparation: 15 minutes
Cooking: 20 minutes
Yield: 4 main-course servings

2 tablespoons olive oil, divided

12 ounces pork loin, thinly sliced

Sea salt to taste

Black pepper to taste

6 cloves garlic, peeled, sliced, and divided

2 tablespoons top-quality balsamic vinegar

12 ounces escarole, trimmed, chopped, washed, and drained

6 tomatoes from a can, seeded and chopped

½ cup dry white wine

1 cup low-sodium chicken broth

8 large Sicilian olives, pitted and chopped

¼ cup fresh basil

1 pound fresh pappardelle

4 ounces Blue Castello or another creamy blue cheese

1. Bring a large pot of water to a boil. Heat 1 tablespoon of the olive oil in a wok over high heat. Sprinkle the pork with sea salt and black pepper. When the oil is hot, carefully place the pork in the pan. Sear the pork, stirring it 2 or 3 times.

2. Move the pork to one side of the wok. Add 3 cloves of the garlic to the wok and cook for 20 seconds. Stir the pork and garlic together and cook for 15 seconds. Add the vinegar to the pan and cook for 30 seconds. Transfer the pork to a plate.

3. Heat the remaining tablespoon of oil in the wok over high heat. Add the remaining garlic to the pan and cook for 30 seconds. Add the escarole to the pan and cook for 1 minute. Add the tomatoes to the pan and cook for 30 seconds.

4. Add the wine to the pan and cook for 30 seconds. Add the chicken broth to the pan and bring to a boil. Reduce the heat and simmer until the escarole is tender.

5. Add olives and basil to the sauce. Stir in pork. Remove the pot from the heat and season with sea salt and black pepper.

6. Add sea salt to the boiling water, followed by the pasta. Cook until tender, approximately 4 minutes. Drain the pasta and add it to the sauce.

7. Cook the pasta and sauce together over low heat for 2 minutes. Divide the pasta among 4 plates and garnish with blue cheese.

Linguine with Corn, Cilantro, and Tofu

Orange-flavored tofu and a sharp-tasting lime sauce are the stand-out flavors in this meal. Corn and Parmesan cheese are good sources of calcium.

Preparation: 15 minutes
Cooking: 10 minutes
Yield: 4 main-course servings

Sea salt to taste
1 pound linguine
2 tablespoons olive oil, divided
1 pound firm tofu, cut into small cubes
⅓ cup fresh orange juice
6 cloves garlic, peeled and sliced
1 red bell pepper, cored and diced
3 ears fresh corn, kernels removed
1 cup low-sodium chicken broth
1 tomato, diced
4 scallions, trimmed and thinly sliced
Juice from 4 limes
½ cup cilantro, chopped
Black pepper to taste
4 tablespoons grated Parmesan cheese

1. Bring a large pot of water to a boil. Add sea salt, followed by the pasta.

2. Heat 1 tablespoon of the olive oil in a wok over high heat. When the oil is hot, add the tofu. Cook the tofu until golden, stirring several times. Add the orange juice and cook the tofu for 1 more minute. Transfer the tofu to a plate and set aside.

3. Heat the remaining olive oil in the wok over medium heat. Add the garlic to the oil and cook 45 seconds. Add the bell pepper to the pan and sprinkle with sea salt. Cook the pepper for 2 minutes, stirring often. Raise the heat to high.

4. Add the corn to the pan and continue cooking and stirring the ingredients for another minute.

5. Add the chicken broth to the pan and bring to a boil. Add the tomato and scallions to the pan. Reduce the heat to

low and stir in the lime juice and cilantro. Season with sea salt and black pepper.

6. Drain the pasta and add it to the sauce. Cook the sauce and pasta together for 2 minutes. Divide the pasta among 4 plates and garnish with the tofu and Parmesan cheese.

Penne with Navy Beans, Greens, and Goat Cheese

Preparation: 15 minutes
Cooking: 25 minutes
Yield: 4 main-course servings

The combination of beans and pasta is a traditional Italian speciality. The beans are an excellent source of fiber. This dish is rich in calcium from the beans, greens, and cheese. Tip: *The tomato-mushroom sauce through step 4 can be prepared a day in advance and refrigerated.*

1 tablespoon extra-virgin olive oil
6 cloves garlic, peeled and sliced
1 pound button mushrooms, sliced
Sea salt to taste
½ cup red wine
1 28-ounce can whole tomatoes, drained and chopped
1 pound penne
1 cup pasta-cooking water
½ pound escarole, trimmed, chopped, washed, and drained
1 large bunch arugula, chopped, washed, and drained
Black pepper to taste
1 15-ounce can Great Northern or navy beans, drained and rinsed
6 ounces goat cheese, room temperature

1. Bring a large pot of water to a boil. Heat the olive oil in a Dutch oven over low heat. Add the garlic to the oil and cook until soft and fragrant, stirring occasionally.

2. Raise the heat to high and add the mushrooms to the Dutch oven. Sprinkle with sea salt and cook until soft and all of their liquid has evaporated. Add the wine and simmer until it has evaporated, approximately 2 minutes.

3. Add the tomatoes to the Dutch oven and bring the sauce to a boil. Reduce the heat to low and simmer the tomatoes for 10 minutes, stirring them often.

4. Add sea salt to the boiling water, followed by the pasta. Cook the pasta until tender. Reserve 1 cup of the pasta cooking water and drain the pasta.

5. Raise the heat to high under the tomatoes and add the pasta-cooking water to them. Add the escarole to the Dutch oven and cook for 3 minutes. Add the arugula and cook the sauce for 2 minutes. Season with sea salt and black pepper.

6. Reduce the heat to low and stir the beans into the sauce. Add the cooked pasta to the sauce and stir over low heat for 2 minutes.

7. Divide the pasta among 4 shallow bowls and garnish with goat cheese.

Arugula

Once considered a specialty green, arugula or rocket is now widely available. Wonderful raw or cooked, the smaller leaves will add a sharp taste to a green salad; the larger leaves are peppery and are best cooked until they just wilt. This versatile vegetable pairs well with mild-flavored greens and creamy cheeses, such as goat's milk and fresh mozzarella.

Arugula tends to be sandy. Swirl it around in a sinkful of cold water and dry it thoroughly before using it in a recipe.

Pizza

Preparation: 2 hours (includes dough preparation)
Cooking: 12 minutes
Yield: 4 main-course servings

With this recipe, you can have your estrogen and eat your pizza, too. When the idea for this recipe was suggested, we were initially skeptical. Were we taking this soy and flaxseed stuff too far? Could we develop recipes for estrogen-laced pizza dough and toppings that would actually taste good? We did, and they taste great.

DOUGH

1 cup soy milk, warmed (110° F)
1 tablespoon brown-rice syrup
2½ teaspoons active dry yeast
½ cup flaxseed, ground
2 cups unbleached flour plus additional flour for kneading
1 teaspoon sea salt
Olive oil for greasing the bowl and sheet pan

TOPPING SUGGESTIONS

1. Soy mozzarella and tomato sauce
2. Cooked spinach, garlic, extra-virgin olive, and Parmesan cheese
3. Roasted bell peppers, cooked mushrooms, tomato sauce, and soy mozzarella

1. Combine the soy milk, brown-rice syrup, and yeast in a bowl. Allow the mixture to proof for 10 minutes.

2. Combine the flaxseed, flour, and sea salt in a large mixing bowl. Slowly stir in the soy milk mixture. Continue stirring until a dough forms.

3. Turn the dough onto a lightly floured surface. Knead for 10 minutes or until smooth and elastic. Add only enough flour to prevent the dough from sticking to the work surface.

4. Lightly oil a large bowl. Place the dough in the bowl and turn to coat the entire surface evenly. Cover the bowl with plastic wrap and place in a warm and draft-free place to rise. Allow the dough to rise for 1½ hours or until it has doubled in bulk.

5. Prepare the topping.

6. Heat the oven to 450°F.

7. To shape the pizza, deflate the dough and form it into a round ball. Roll the dough onto a lightly floured surface and shape it into a rectangle about 1/8-inch thick. Place the dough in a lightly oiled, heavy-duty, 16-inch sheet pan. Cover the pizza with the chosen topping. Bake the pizza for 10 to 12 minutes or until the crust is golden.

Broccoli–Olive Pesto, Pecan, and Goat Cheese Pizza

With tofu in the topping and flaxseed in the crust, you get phytoestrogens from two sources in this recipe as well as a calcium boost from the broccoli and cheese.

Preparation: 2 hours (includes dough preparation)
Cooking: 12 minutes
Yield: 4 main-course servings

¼ **cup pecans, coarsely chopped**

1 **cup water**

Sea salt to taste

4 **cups broccoli florets (reserve the stems for another use)**

1 **small clove garlic, peeled and minced**

¼ **cup pine nuts**

8 **Kalamata olives, pitted**

4 **ounces silken tofu**

⅓ **cup grated Romano cheese**

Black pepper to taste

Pizza dough (see page 208), ready to roll out

4 **ounces goat cheese**

1. Place the pecans in a small skillet over very low heat. Toast them until fragrant and no longer raw tasting, shaking the pan often, approximately 12 minutes.

2. Meanwhile, heat the oven to 450°F. Place the water in a medium-sized pot over high heat. Bring the water to a boil

and add a dash of sea salt. Add the broccoli florets to the water and steam until tender, approximately 4 minutes. Drain the broccoli and cool it under running water.

3. Squeeze the broccoli to remove any excess moisture. Transfer it to the work bowl of a food processor fitted with a metal blade. Add the garlic, pine nuts, olives, and tofu to the work bowl. Process until a smooth pesto forms. Stir in the Romano cheese and season the pesto with sea salt and black pepper.

4. Roll out the dough and place it in a lightly oiled, heavy-duty, 16-inch sheet pan. Spread the pesto evenly on the dough. There might be extra. Dot the pizza with the goat cheese and sprinkle on the pecans.

5. Bake the pizza for 10 to 12 minutes or until the crust is golden. Remove it from the oven and slice it. Accompany with Romaine Salad with Garlic Croutons and Balsamic Vinegar (see page 166).

Tomato Pesto and Portobello Mushroom Pizza

Preparation: 2 hours (includes dough preparation)
Cooking: 12 minutes
Yield: 4 main-course servings

Pizza can be heart-healthy if you use vegetarian toppings. Fresh and dried tomatoes, fresh basil, and pine nuts create an intensely tomato-flavored pesto. Earthy portobello mushrooms and mild-flavored soy mozzarella add just the right contrasts to this pizza.

½ **cup dried tomatoes**
1 **cup boiling water**
4 **teaspoons olive oil, divided**
6 **cloves garlic, peeled, sliced, and divided**
1 **cup dried tomato–soaking water**
2 **cups fresh tomatoes, peeled, seeded, and chopped or 2 cups canned whole tomatoes, drained, and chopped**

4 ounces silken tofu

¼ cup pine nuts

⅓ cup fresh basil

Sea salt to taste

Black pepper to taste

8 ounces portobello mushrooms, stems removed (reserve them for a stock) and caps sliced

Pizza dough (see page 208), ready to roll out

6 ounces soy mozzarella, grated or sliced

1. Heat the oven to 450°F. Place the dried tomatoes in a bowl and pour the water on them. Allow them to soften for 10 minutes. Drain and reserve their soaking water.

2. Meanwhile, heat 2 teaspoons of the olive oil in a Dutch oven over low heat. Add 4 cloves of garlic and cook until soft. Raise the heat to high and add the tomato-soaking water. Add the tomatoes and bring the sauce to a boil.

3. Reduce the heat and simmer the sauce, stirring occasionally, until all of the liquid has evaporated, approximately 15 minutes.

4. Transfer the sauce to the work bowl of a food processor fitted with a metal blade. Add the softened tomatoes, tofu, pine nuts, and basil to the bowl. Process until a smooth pesto forms. Season with sea salt and black pepper.

5. Heat the remaining 2 teaspoons of olive oil in a skillet over high heat. When the oil is hot, add the remaining garlic to the pan and cook it for 15 seconds. Add the mushrooms to the pan and sprinkle with sea salt. Cook the mushrooms, stirring often, until soft, approximately 7 minutes.

6. Roll out the dough and place it in a lightly oiled, heavy-duty, 16-inch sheet pan. Spread the pesto evenly on the dough. There might be extra. Sprinkle on the mushrooms and mozzarella.

7. Bake the pizza for 10 to 12 minutes or until the crust is golden. Remove it from the oven and slice it. Accompany with Creamy Caesar Salad (see page 173).

Chapter 15

Vegetarian Dishes

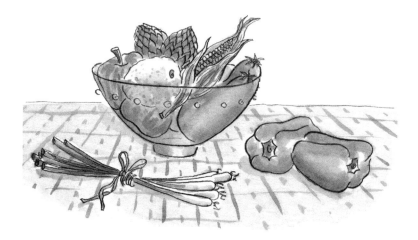

Soy is a vegetarian superfood. If you are a vegetarian, or if you are like us and have an occasional serving of poultry, fish, or meat to accompany a well-balanced diet, soy foods in menopause are a superb protein source. Soy is one of the principal sources of phytoestrogens, so it is important to eat soy regularly.

The highest hurdle facing vegetarians is consuming top-quality protein. A varied diet is rich in dried beans, peas, whole-grain breads, pasta, and rice. Soy is arguably the best nonmeat protein source of all and in menopause has the added bonus of increasing the phytoestrogen content of your diet. In addition to getting enough protein, vegetarians need to pay special attention to the foods they eat in order to ingest adequate amounts of B vitamins, iron, calcium, and zinc.

You do not need to eat complex or elaborate vegetarian meals in order to meet your nutritional needs in menopause. Some vegetarian dishes, such as those focused on pasta, are simple to prepare. Virtually endless combinations of pastas, vegetables, and cheeses can be used to make delectable meals. The Pasta and Pizza chapter in this book has several examples.

However, taking a block of tofu or tempeh and turning it into a tasty and satisfying meal can be a challenge. Unlike meat, poultry, and fish, soy products such as tofu and tempeh can't stand on their own. While they can be the star of the show, they need a strong supporting cast. Their versatility, practicality, and ability to absorb flavors lend a unique texture to a meal. That function is most evident when they are combined with vegetables, nuts, grains, cheese, and robust seasonings.

The next time you have vegetarians over for dinner and are not certain what to serve, don't fret. Surprise them with Curried Chickpeas, Tofu, and Arugula. The intense flavor of the sauce and interesting combination of textures is sure to win them over. Or try a warm Salad of Grilled Tomatoes, Tofu, Portobello Mushrooms, and Radicchio. And with firm and silken tofu in these recipes, they are loaded with phytoestrogens.

Burritos are a popular fast food now, but the problem for vegetarians is that they usually are based upon chicken, beef, or pork, so you are left with a filling of only rice and beans. While rice and beans are a healthful choice, why not add a soy source to the filling to make them even better? You can make delicious and estrogen-rich burritos at home with our Tempeh and Vegetable Burritos.

Although preparing vegetarian meals sometimes can be more time consuming than preparing meat-based ones, they also can be more practical. Many vegetarian meals can be made entirely ahead of time without any loss of flavor or texture. In fact, they taste even better the following day. Most meat-based meals have to be made "to order" or they have that reheated flavor. Our delicious Acorn Squash Stuffed with Brown Rice, Tofu, and Dried Cranberries and our Gratin of Potatoes, Chard, and Roasted Peppers are make-ahead favorites, whose flavor is enhanced by a day of sitting in the refrigerator.

Whether you are a strict vegetarian or just enjoy preparing and eating vegetarian food, soy as the main attraction will make your meals unique, great tasting, and rich in protein and phytoestrogen.

Acorn Squash Stuffed with Brown Rice, Tofu, and Dried Cranberries

Preparation: 20 minutes
Cooking: 1 hour
Yield: 6 main-course servings

This meal is as nutritious as it is beautiful and delicious. Tofu, brown rice, dried cranberries, and soy cheddar ensure that it is packed with phytoestrogens and fiber. Tip: *The entire recipe can be prepared a day in advance. Heat the squash in a 350°F oven for approximately 25 minutes or until the interior is hot.*

3 medium acorn squash, halved and seeded
Olive oil for rubbing
Sea salt to taste
Black pepper to taste
3 cups water
1⅓ cups brown rice
⅓ pound dried cranberries
1 tablespoon canola oil
12 ounces firm tofu, cut into small cubes
1 medium leek, washed, trimmed, and thinly sliced
Juice of 2 juice oranges
⅓ cup walnuts, coarsely chopped and lightly toasted
½ cup cilantro, chopped
6 ounces soy cheddar, grated

1. Heat the oven to 425°F.
2. Rub the flesh of each squash half with olive oil and sprin-

kle with sea salt and black pepper. Place the squash halves, flesh side down, on a heavy baking sheet. Roast until tender, approximately 40 minutes. Remove from the oven and set aside. Do not turn the oven off.

3. While the squash halves are baking, bring the water to a boil in a medium-sized pan and add a dash of sea salt. Stir the brown rice into the water, cover the pan, and reduce the heat to a simmer. Cook the rice until tender and all of the water has evaporated, approximately 45 minutes. During the last 10 minutes, sprinkle the cranberries onto the top of the rice.

4. While the squash and rice are cooking, heat the canola oil in a wok over high heat. When it is hot, add the tofu. Cook the tofu until golden, stirring several times. Add the leeks to the wok and stir continually until soft. Add the orange juice to the wok and cook the ingredients until the juice has been absorbed. Stir in the walnuts and cilantro and remove the wok from the heat.

5. Stir the cooked brown rice and cranberries into the tofu mixture and allow the mixture to cool for 5 minutes. Season with sea salt and black pepper.

6. Fill the cavity of each squash half with the rice mixture and sprinkle the stuffed squash with the cheese.

7. Return the squash to the oven and bake until the cheese has melted, approximately 10 minutes.

Broccoli-and-Mushroom-Stuffed Potatoes

Baked and filled potatoes often contain butter and other fat-laden ingredients. This version is made creamy by the combination of silken tofu and goat cheese. The potatoes are rich in calcium, phytoestrogens, and fiber. Tips: *This recipe can be prepared a day in advance. The following day sprinkle the potatoes with the almonds and cheddar and bake them in a 375°F oven until they are hot.*

Preparation: 15 minutes
Cooking: 1¼ hours
Yield: 4 main-course servings

4 large baking potatoes, scrubbed

⅓ cup almonds

2 teaspoons olive oil

3 cloves garlic, peeled and sliced

12 ounces white mushrooms, sliced

2 cups water

Sea salt to taste

1¼ pounds broccoli, trimmed, stems peeled and sliced,
   florets separated

8 ounces silken tofu

4 ounces goat cheese

Black pepper to taste

4 ounces soy cheddar, grated or sliced

1. Heat the oven to 400°F. Place the potatoes on an oven rack and bake until soft, approximately 1 hour. Remove them from the oven and allow to cool. Do not turn off the oven.

2. While the potatoes are baking, place the almonds in a small skillet and toast over low heat until golden, shaking the pan several times. Set the almonds aside.

3. Heat the oil in a skillet over medium-high heat. Add the garlic and cook for 40 seconds. Add the mushrooms and cook until soft. Set the mushrooms aside.

4. Bring the water to a boil in a Dutch oven. Add a dash of sea salt to the water, followed by the broccoli. Cover the pot and steam the broccoli until tender. Drain it and cool it under running water. Transfer the broccoli to the work bowl of a food processor fitted with the metal blade.

5. Place the tofu and goat cheese in the processor and process until smooth. Set the mixture aside.

6. Slice the potatoes in half and scoop their flesh into a mixing bowl. Mash the flesh with a fork. Add the mushrooms and tofu-broccoli mixture to the potatoes and combine them. Season with sea salt and black pepper.

7. Fill the potato jackets with the filling. Garnish each potato with the almonds and cheddar. Place the potatoes on a baking tray and bake for 20 minutes.

8. Divide the potatoes among 4 plates and accompany with a mesclun salad.

Balsamic Vinegar

Once you have tasted the sweet, rich, and intensely fruity flavor of a top-quality balsamic vinegar, you never again will use the inferior mass-produced variety. Balsamic vinegar is produced in Modena, Italy, from the juice of Trebbiano grapes. It is aged in barrels of a variety of woods, including oak, cherry, and juniper, from a period of six years to several decades. If you searched enough, it would be possible to locate a 100-year-old balsamic. Much easier to locate and afford is a 10-year-old bottle, which will have a smoothness and sweetness that a younger bottle will lack.

Balsamic vinegar makes a wonderful vinaigrette and adds a zip to fresh fruits. Drizzled on tofu, meat, or poultry and cooked for 30 seconds, it adds an unexpected sweet flavor to a dish.

Salad of Grilled Tomatoes, Tofu, Portobello Mushrooms, and Radicchio

Prepare this salad the next time you grill. Radicchio most often is used uncooked in a salad where it is prized for its bitterness and crunch, but here we have grilled it, along with tofu, portobello mushrooms, and tomatoes. Grilling radicchio tames its sharp taste and adds a wonderful contrast to the lemony tofu and hearty mushrooms. You will not miss grilled steak with this delicious and healthful salad. Tip: *It is necessary to plan ahead to prepare this salad. The tofu needs to marinate for 2 hours.*

Preparation: 20 minutes (2 hours for tofu)
Cooking: 15 minutes
Yield: 6 side-dish servings

TOFU MARINADE

Juice from 2 lemons
2 tablespoons extra-virgin olive oil
2 tablespoons fresh rosemary, finely chopped
Sea salt to taste
Black pepper to taste
1 pound firm tofu sliced into 1-inch-thick triangles

DRESSING

2 tablespoons top-quality balsamic vinegar
1 teaspoon Dijon mustard
3 tablespoons extra-virgin olive oil
2 tablespoons fresh basil, snipped
Sea salt to taste
Black pepper to taste

REMAINING INGREDIENTS

4 tomatoes, cored and halved
3 portobello mushrooms, stems removed
1 medium head radicchio, quartered
Extra-virgin olive oil for drizzling
Sea salt to taste
Black pepper to taste
4 ounces goat cheese, room temperature

1. To prepare the tofu marinade, whisk together the lemon juice, olive oil, and rosemary in a shallow bowl. Season with sea salt and black pepper. Place the tofu in the marinade and turn several times. Marinate the tofu for 2 hours, turning once.

2. Prepare a hardwood charcoal fire. While the fire is ashing over, prepare the dressing by whisking together the vinegar and mustard. Drizzle in the olive oil and whisk the dressing until it emulsifies. Stir in the basil and season the dressing with sea salt and black pepper. Set the dressing aside.

3. Drizzle the tomatoes, mushrooms, and radicchio with olive oil and sprinkle with sea salt and black pepper.

4. Grill the tomatoes, turning often, until well marked.

Transfer them to a plate to cool. Grill the mushrooms, turning several times, until very soft. Transfer to the plate to cool. Grill the radicchio, turning often, until it is wilted. Transfer to the plate to cool. Remove the tofu from the marinade and grill until grill marks appear on each side. Transfer it to the plate to cool.

5. When the vegetables and tofu are cool enough to handle, slice into medium-sized pieces and place on a large serving platter. Dot the salad with goat cheese and drizzle with the dressing. Serve at once.

Tofu and Chickpea Patties with a Yogurt-Chili Sauce

These tofu and chickpea patties are unique and delicious. The cool and tangy yogurt-chili sauce is the perfect complement. The tofu in both the chickpea patties and the yogurt sauce provides a great amount of phytoestrogens. Tip: *The tofu mixture (without the egg) and the yogurt sauce can be prepared a day in advance. In fact, the sauce tastes better on the second day. An overnight chill allows the flavors to develop fully.*

Preparation: 25 minutes
Cooking: 20 minutes
Chilling: 2 hours
Yield: 4 main-course servings

YOGURT SAUCE

- 1–2 jalapeño peppers, seeded and chopped
- 1 cup plain nonfat yogurt
- 4 ounces silken tofu, chopped
- 1 clove garlic, peeled and finely chopped
- 1 shallot, peeled and chopped
- 3 scallions, trimmed and sliced
- 1 medium tomato, cored and diced
- Juice from one lemon
- ⅓ cup cilantro, chopped
- Sea salt to taste
- Black pepper to taste

Tofu Chickpea Patties

2 teaspoons olive oil

3 cloves garlic, peeled and finely chopped

1 medium onion, diced

1 medium carrot, scraped and finely chopped

Sea salt to taste

2 teaspoons curry powder

4 scallions, trimmed and thinly sliced

⅓ cup flat-leaf parsley, chopped

1 15-ounce can chickpeas, drained and rinsed

12 ounces firm tofu, coarsely chopped

½ cup breadcrumbs

2 tablespoons tahini

Black pepper to taste

1 egg

2–3 tablespoons canola oil

1. Place the peppers, yogurt, silken tofu, garlic, shallot, scallions, tomato, lemon juice, and cilantro in the bowl of a food processor fitted with a metal blade. Puree the mixture. Season with sea salt and black pepper. Cover and refrigerate for at least 2 hours.

2. Heat the oven to 400°F. Heat the olive oil in a large skillet over low heat. Add the garlic to the skillet and cook until soft and fragrant. Add the onion to the skillet and cook until soft.

3. Raise the heat slightly and add the carrot to the skillet. Sprinkle with sea salt. Cover the pot and steam the vegetables for 5 minutes, stirring occasionally. Add curry powder and cook for 2 more minutes.

4. Add the scallions and parsley to the skillet. Cover the skillet and set aside.

5. Place the chickpeas, tofu, breadcrumbs, and tahini in the work bowl of a food processor fitted with a metal blade. Process until a slightly chunky consistency is achieved. Add the cooked vegetables and process until smooth. Season with sea salt and black pepper. Stir the egg into the mixture.

6. Form the mixture into 16 patties.

7. Pour the canola oil onto a heavy baking tray. Place the tray in the oven. Allow the oil to get hot. Remove the tray from the oven and place the patties on it, tilting the tray to spread the oil evenly. Return the tray to the oven and bake the patties until their bottoms are golden, approximately 10 minutes. Flip the patties and bake for 5 to 8 minutes more.

8. Divide the patties among four plates and drizzle the yogurt sauce on each. Accompany with a green salad and rustic bread.

Cooking Dried Herbs and Spices
Gently cooking dried herbs and spices before adding any liquid ingredients to a recipe mellows their bitter taste and brings out their unique flavors. For example, a quick tomato sauce usually contains olive oil, garlic, onion, dried basil, oregano, and thyme. If the herbs are cooked for 1 or 2 minutes with the onion, their flavor will be sweeter and more intense. If they are added after the tomatoes, their flavor will be raw and not as distinctive. The same reasoning applies to dried spices. Briefly cooking curry powder with garlic and fresh ginger results in a smooth and sweet-tasting sauce.

Gratin of Potatoes, Chard, and Roasted Peppers

Traditional gratins contain a great deal of butter, cream, and cheese, making them high in saturated fat and calories. This version is lighter and phytoestrogen rich, containing soy milk and silken tofu. It is also rich in fiber. Tip: *This recipe can be assembled earlier in the day and placed in the oven 40 minutes before serving time.*

Preparation: 20 minutes
Cooking: 45 minutes
Yield: 4 main-course servings

2 tablespoons olive oil, divided
12 ounces silken tofu
4 ounces goat cheese
4 medium Yukon Gold, Yellow Finn, or russet potatoes,
   scrubbed and thinly sliced
2 cups soy milk
Sea salt to taste
Black pepper to taste
5 cloves garlic, sliced
1 pound Swiss chard, chopped, washed, and drained
3 roasted red bell peppers, thinly sliced
1 15-ounce can chickpeas, drained and rinsed
2½ cups fresh breadcrumbs (see page 275)

1. Heat the oven to 400°F. Spread 1 tablespoon of the olive oil in a 10-inch cast-iron skillet.

2. Combine the tofu and goat cheese in the work bowl of a food processor fitted with a metal blade and puree the ingredients. Set the mixture aside.

3. Place the potatoes in a saucepan and cover them with soy milk. Season with sea salt and black pepper. Bring the mixture to a boil, reduce the heat, and simmer until the potatoes are just tender, approximately 10 minutes. Drain and allow to cool.

4. While the potatoes are cooking, heat the remaining tablespoon of olive oil in a wok over high heat. Add the garlic and cook for 30 seconds. Add the chard to the wok, cover it, and cook the chard until tender, stirring often. If necessary, add water to the chard to prevent it from sticking.

5. Remove the wok from the heat and stir in the roasted bell peppers and chickpeas. Season with sea salt and black pepper.

6. Layer the potatoes, chard mixture, and tofu mixture in the prepared skillet, beginning and ending with the potatoes. Cover the final layer with breadcrumbs.

7. Place the skillet in the oven and bake the gratin until the topping is crusty and the filling hot, approximately 45 minutes. Divide the gratin among 4 plates and serve at once.

Saffron Rice with Baked Garlic and Vegetables

This dish is based upon a recipe from Vince's Spanish grand-mother: Rice in the Oven. This version contains collard greens and chickpeas, both good vegetarian sources of calcium, as well as phytoestrogen-rich tofu.

Preparation: 15 minutes
Cooking: 1 hour
Yield: 4 main-course servings

2 tablespoons extra-virgin olive oil
5 cloves garlic, peeled and sliced
1 onion, peeled and diced
Sea salt to taste
2 medium tomatoes, cored and diced
1 pound firm tofu, cut into small cubes
⅔ teaspoon sweet paprika
4 cups vegetable broth (see page 124) or water
1 15-ounce can chickpeas, drained and rinsed
2 large bulbs garlic, loose skin removed, ¼-inch sliced off the top to expose the raw garlic
¾ pound collard greens, trimmed, washed, and drained
Black pepper to taste
Large pinch of saffron threads
1½ cups short-grain white rice
Reserved saffron liquid
1 14-ounce can artichoke hearts, drained, rinsed, and sliced
1 large potato, peeled and thinly sliced
1 roasted red bell pepper or 1 small jar pimentos, sliced
2 lemons, sliced into wedges

1. Heat the olive oil in a Dutch oven over medium heat. Add the sliced garlic to the pot and cook until soft and fragrant, stirring constantly.

2. Add onion to the pot and sprinkle with sea salt. Cook until soft, stirring often. Add tomatoes, tofu, and paprika to the pot. Cook tomatoes until soft, approximately 3 minutes.

3. Raise the heat to high and add the vegetable broth or water. Bring the liquid to a boil and stir in the chickpeas, whole bulbs of garlic, and collard greens. Reduce the heat to low, cover the pot, and simmer for 15 minutes. Season with sea salt and black pepper.

4. Remove the cover and carefully ladle 4 ounces of the liquid into a small bowl. Crush the saffron threads into the hot liquid and set the bowl aside.

5. Raise the heat to high under the Dutch oven. When the ingredients return to the boil, stir in the rice and the reserved saffron liquid. Stir the artichoke hearts into the pot.

6. Reduce the heat to a low simmer. Scatter the potato slices and roasted bell pepper slices on the rice. Cover the pot and simmer until all of the liquid is absorbed and the rice is tender, approximately 40 minutes.

7. Spoon a portion of the rice onto a plate along with several of the garlic cloves. Accompany with the lemon wedges.

Lentil Stew with Leeks, Potatoes, and Goat Cheese

Preparation: 15 minutes
Cooking: 1 hour
Yield: 4 main-course servings

This rich stew will warm you on a cold winter day. It is very rich in fiber from the lentils. A garnish of crisp potatoes, tofu, and leeks adds flavor and phytoestrogens. Tip: *The stew can be prepared a day in advance. Reheat it over low heat, adding more water to thin it if necessary. Prepare the garnishes just before you serve the stew.*

2 teaspoons canola oil
3 cloves garlic, peeled and sliced
1 onion, peeled and diced
1 rib celery, diced
2 carrots, peeled and diced
Sea salt to taste

1½ cups green lentils, rinsed

4–5 cups chicken or vegetable broth or water

2 medium Yellow Finn potatoes, scrubbed and cubed

2 tablespoons olive oil, divided

Black pepper to taste

1 pound firm tofu, cut into small cubes

2 medium leeks, trimmed, cut in half vertically, washed, and thinly sliced

1 pound spinach, trimmed, chopped, washed, and drained

4 ounces goat cheese, room temperature

1. Heat the canola oil in a Dutch oven over low heat. Add the garlic to the pot and cook until soft and fragrant. Add the onion to the pot and cook until it begins to soften, stirring occasionally.

2. Add the celery, carrots, and a pinch of sea salt to the pot. Raise the heat slightly, cover the pot, and steam for 5 minutes, stirring occasionally.

3. Add the lentils to the pot and cook them for 3 minutes. Raise the heat to high and add the broth or water. Bring the stew to a boil, reduce the heat, and simmer until the lentils are tender, approximately 45 minutes.

4. While the stew is cooking, prepare the garnishes. Heat the oven to 400° F. Place the potato cubes in a bowl, drizzle them with 1 tablespoon of the olive oil, and sprinkle with sea salt and black pepper. Transfer them to a baking tray and roast until golden, approximately 30 minutes. Set them aside.

5. Heat the remaining tablespoon of olive oil in a wok over high heat. When the oil is hot, add the tofu. Cook the tofu until golden, stirring occasionally. Add the leeks to the tofu and sprinkle with sea salt. Cook the leeks until soft, stirring constantly. Set the ingredients aside.

6. When the lentils are tender, stir the spinach into the stew and cook until it wilts. Season with sea salt and black pepper.

7. Ladle the stew into 4 large bowls and garnish with potatoes, the tofu-leek mixture, and a dot of goat cheese. Accompany with rustic bread.

Roasted Squash, Parsnip, Leek, and Tofu Stew

*Preparation: 15
minutes*
Cooking: 55 minutes
*Yield: 6 main-course
servings*

In a traditional stew, meat is the centerpiece with vegetables playing a supporting role. Such a stew always takes several hours of slow cooking to transform a tough cut of meat into a fork-tender delight. We have created a wonderful meatless stew that takes less than an hour to prepare with roasted root vegetables, orange-flavored tofu, and hearty beans as the standout ingredients. The stew is packed with fiber, antioxidants, and phytoestrogens. Tip: If the top layer of the leeks chars, remove and discard it. The remaining leaves will be tender and sweet.

1 butternut squash, peeled, seeded, halved, and sliced into eighths

3 parsnips, peeled, quartered lengthwise and halved

3 carrots, peeled, quartered lengthwise and halved

2 leeks, trimmed, washed, and halved lengthwise

2 red onions, peeled and quartered

4 plum tomatoes, halved

4 tablespoons olive oil, divided

Sea salt to taste

Pepper to taste

4 cloves garlic, peeled and sliced

1 yellow onion, peeled and diced

1 16-ounce can soybeans, drained and rinsed

1 16-ounce can white beans, drained and rinsed

1 28-ounce can whole tomatoes, drained (reserve the juice for another recipe) and chopped

4 cups water

1 pound firm tofu, sliced into small cubes

1 tablespoon sugar

4 tablespoons orange juice

4 tablespoons fresh oregano, chopped

1. Heat the oven to 400°F. Place the squash, parsnips, carrots, leeks, onions, and tomatoes in a single layer on 1 large or 2 smaller heavy baking trays. Drizzle with 2 tablespoons of olive oil and sprinkle with sea salt and black pepper. Transfer the tray to the oven and roast the vegetables until they are slightly caramelized and tender, approximately 50 minutes.

2. Meanwhile, heat another tablespoon of olive oil in a Dutch oven over low heat. Add the garlic to the pot and cook until soft and fragrant. Add the onion to the pot and cook until soft, stirring occasionally.

3. Add the soybeans and white beans into the pot. Stir the beans and cook the ingredients for 2 minutes. Raise the heat to high and add the tomatoes to the pot.

4. Add the water to the pot and bring the broth to a boil. Reduce the heat and simmer for 25 minutes. Season with sea salt and black pepper.

5. While the vegetables are roasting and the broth is simmering, heat the remaining 1 tablespoon of olive oil in a well-seasoned wok over high heat. When the oil is hot, add the tofu. Cook the tofu until golden, approximately 4 minutes, stirring several times. Sprinkle the tofu with the sugar and drizzle it with the orange juice. Cook the tofu for 30 seconds more and then set it aside.

6. When the vegetables are tender, divide them among 6 bowls. Divide the tofu among the bowls. Stir the oregano into the broth. Ladle the broth into each bowl and serve at once.

Curried Chickpeas, Tofu, and Arugula

This Indian-inspired dish is rich in antioxidants and fiber and low in fat, making it very heart-healthy. Both the cubed firm tofu and the silken tofu in the recipe provide plenty of phytoestrogens. Serve it with brown rice or Basmati Rice with Almonds and Raisins (see page 277).

Preparation: 15 minutes
Cooking: 30 minutes
Yield: 4 main-course servings

1 tablespoon canola oil

4 cloves garlic, peeled and sliced

1 1-inch piece gingerroot, peeled and minced

1 onion, peeled and diced

2 carrots, peeled and diced

1 rib celery, diced

Sea salt to taste

12 ounces firm tofu, sliced into small cubes

1 15-ounce can chickpeas, drained and rinsed

1 heaping tablespoon curry powder

½ teaspoon ground cumin

½ teaspoon ground coriander

¼ teaspoon nutmeg

¼ teaspoon ground cinnamon

3 cups water

1 28-ounce can whole tomatoes, drained and chopped

½ pound arugula, trimmed, washed, drained, and chopped

Black pepper to taste

8 ounces silken tofu, pureed

1. Heat the canola oil in a Dutch oven over low heat. Add the garlic and gingerroot and cook until soft and fragrant. Add the onion and cook until soft, stirring occasionally.

2. Add the carrots and celery and sprinkle with sea salt. Cook the ingredients for 7 minutes, stirring occasionally. Add the tofu, chickpeas, curry, cumin, coriander, nutmeg, and cinnamon. Cook for 3 minutes, stirring often.

3. Raise the heat to high and add the water. Add the tomatoes and bring to a boil.

4. Reduce the heat and simmer for 20 minutes, stirring occasionally. Add the arugula to the pot and cook until it wilts, stirring constantly.

5. Remove the pot from the heat and season with sea salt and black pepper. Stir in the silken tofu.

6. Divide the chickpeas among 4 plates and serve at once.

Tofu and Vegetables in a Peanut Sauce

This vegetarian dish is rich and delicious. It has a double dose of phytoestrogens, containing both miso and silken tofu. Broccoli is an excellent vegetarian source of calcium and is rich in antioxidants. Tips: *The sauce can be prepared and the vegetables steamed a day in advance. We recommend using fresh ground peanut butter in this sauce. If it is unavailable, substitute a brand that is free of additives.*

Preparation: 15 minutes
Cooking: 35 minutes
Yield: 4 main-course servings

SAUCE

  1 cup water
  2 tablespoons dark miso
  ½ cup natural peanut butter
  3 tablespoons molasses
  1 tablespoon honey
  2 tablespoons cider vinegar
  3 tablespoons shoyu or tamari
  4 ounces silken tofu

REMAINING INGREDIENTS

  4½ cups water, divided
  1½ cups sushi rice
  Sea salt to taste
  1 large carrot, peeled and sliced into ⅓-inch disks
  1 pound broccoli, trimmed, stems peeled and sliced into
    ⅓-inch disks florets cut into 2-inch pieces
  1 tablespoon canola oil
  1 1-inch piece gingerroot, peeled and minced
  1 red bell pepper, seeded and sliced
  1 zucchini, sliced
  12 ounces firm tofu, sliced into small cubes

1. To prepare the sauce, place the water in a saucepan and bring to a boil. Remove from the heat and whisk in the miso.

Whisk in the peanut butter, molasses, honey, vinegar, and shoyu. Whisk the sauce until smooth. Place the tofu in the work bowl of a food processor fitted with a metal blade. Puree the tofu and stir into the peanut butter mixture. Set the sauce aside.

2. To complete the recipe, bring 3 cups of the water to a boil in a saucepan. Stir the rice into the water and return the water to a boil. Reduce the heat, cover the pot, and simmer the rice until tender, approximately 25 minutes.

3. While the rice is cooking, bring the remaining 1½ cups of water to a boil in a Dutch oven. Add a dash of sea salt to the water. Place the carrot disks in the water and cover the pot. Steam for 2 minutes. Add the broccoli and steam for 5 minutes longer or until the broccoli is tender. Drain the vegetables and run them under cold water. Set the vegetables aside.

4. Heat the oil in a wok over high heat. When the oil is hot, add the gingerroot to the wok. Cook for 30 seconds. Add the bell pepper and zucchini and cook until the bell pepper begins to soften. Add the tofu and cook for 3 more minutes.

5. Add the steamed vegetables to the wok and cook the ingredients until hot, stirring often. Add the peanut sauce to the wok and simmer until it begins to bubble.

6. Divide the rice among four plates. Spoon the tofu and vegetables onto each plate and serve immediately.

Sesame–Soy Tofu and Vegetables

Preparation: 30 minutes
Cooking: 10 minutes
Yield: 4 main-course servings

Ketchup and Dijon mustard in an otherwise Asian-inspired sauce? It sounds odd, but they do produce a delectable sauce. The tofu provides a dose of phytoestrogens, while the variety of vegetables are rich in antioxidants. The dish is low in calories and very heart-healthy. Tips: *Quite a bit of preparation is involved in this recipe, but once you have things in order, it moves quickly. The vegetables can be steamed and the sauce prepared a day in advance. Also, linguine or Asian-style noodles, such as udon (12–16 ounces), can be substituted for the rice. As with all noodle dishes, toss the cooked noodles with the tofu and vegetables for 2 minutes over low heat in the wok.*

SAUCE

- 1 teaspoon sesame oil
- 1 tablespoon ketchup
- 1 tablespoon Dijon mustard
- 4 tablespoons shoyu or tamari
- 3 tablespoons oyster sauce
- 1 teaspoon sugar
- 1 cup vegetable-steaming water (see below)

RICE

- 3 cups water
- 1½ cups sushi rice or short-grain white rice

REMAINING INGREDIENTS

- 1 cup water
- Sea salt to taste
- 3 carrots, peeled and cut into 1-inch pieces
- 2 ribs celery, cut into 1-inch pieces
- 1 head broccoli, trimmed and cut into 2-inch pieces
- 2 tablespoons canola oil, divided
- 12 ounces firm tofu, cut into small cubes
- 4 cloves garlic, peeled and sliced
- ½-inch piece gingerroot, peeled and sliced
- 1 portobello mushroom, stemmed and sliced
- 1 Italian or 2 Japanese eggplants, cut into 1-inch pieces
- 4 tablespoons soy nuts

1. To make the sauce, combine the sesame oil, ketchup, mustard, shoyu, oyster sauce, and sugar in a bowl and whisk the ingredients well. You will add the vegetable-steaming water later. Set the sauce aside.

2. To make the rice, bring the water to a boil in a saucepan.

Stir in the rice. Bring the water back to a boil. Cover the pot and reduce the heat to a low simmer. Cook the rice until all of the liquid has been absorbed, approximately 25 minutes. Set the rice aside.

3. While the rice is cooking, bring the water to a boil in a Dutch oven and add a dash of sea salt. Place the carrots and celery in the water and cover the pot. Steam the vegetables for 2 minutes. Add the broccoli to the pot and for 5 minutes longer. Drain the vegetables, reserving their steaming water. Spray the vegetables with cold water to stop their cooking and set aside. Pour the reserved water into the sauce.

4. Heat 1 tablespoon of the oil in a wok over high heat. When the oil is hot, carefully place the tofu in the wok in a single layer. Cook until it is golden, stirring 3 times. Remove the tofu from the wok and set aside.

5. Heat the remaining oil in the wok over high heat. Add the garlic and gingerroot to the wok and cook for 30 seconds. Add the mushroom and eggplant to the wok and cook until they begin to soften. Stir in the tofu and steamed vegetables to the wok.

6. Whisk the sauce and pour it into the wok. Cook the ingredients for 2 minutes.

7. Transfer the meal to a large platter and garnish with the soy nuts. Divide the rice among four plates and serve the tofu and vegetables family-style.

Orange–Sesame Tofu with Broccoli and Bok Choy

Preparation: 15 minutes
Cooking: 35 minutes
Yield: 4 main-course servings

Tofu takes on the taste of whatever sauce you prepare it in. This orange-sesame sauce is refreshing and delicious. Both broccoli and bok choy are rich in calcium, as is tofu, which makes this dish rich in both phytoestrogens and calcium, a perfect menopause meal. Tips: An efficient method for juicing citrus fruits without using any kitchen utensils is to squeeze one-half of a fruit into the closed fingers of your other hand. Also, when removing the zest from citrus fruits, avoid the white pith, as it will add an unpleasant bitterness to the dish.

5 cups water, divided

Sea salt to taste

6 strips wakami (a sea vegetable), optional

1 bunch broccoli, trimmed and sliced into large florets

1½ cups sushi rice

Juice from 3 juice oranges

2 tablespoons shoyu sauce or tamari

1 tablespoon sesame oil

1 teaspoon sugar

1 tablespoon orange zest

Vegetable-steaming water

2 tablespoons canola oil, divided

1 pound firm tofu, cut into small cubes

1 red bell pepper, seeded and julienned

1 zucchini, julienned

**8 ounces bok choy, trimmed, stems sliced diagonally into
  ¾-inch-thick pieces and leaves coarsely chopped**

2 cloves garlic, peeled and sliced

1 1-inch piece gingerroot, peeled and chopped

4 tablespoons soy nuts

1. Place 2 cups of water in a Dutch oven. Bring the water to a boil and add a dash of sea salt. Add the wakami to the water, cover the pot, and steam it for 15 minutes. Add the broccoli to the pot and steam for 5 minutes longer. Strain the vegetables and reserve their steaming water. Rinse the vegetables under cold water and set them aside.

2. While the vegetables are steaming, bring the remaining 3 cups of water to a boil in a medium pan. Add the rice to the water. Cover the pot, reduce the heat, and simmer the rice until all of the water has been absorbed, approximately 20 minutes. Set the rice aside.

3. While the rice is cooking, prepare the sauce. Whisk together the orange juice, shoyu, sesame oil, sugar, orange zest, and vegetable-steaming water.

4. Heat 1 tablespoon of the canola oil in a wok over high heat. When the oil is hot, carefully place the tofu in a single layer in the wok. Sear the tofu until golden, stirring 3 or 4 times. Add 5 tablespoons of the sauce to the wok and continue cooking until the sauce has been absorbed, approximately 1 minute. Remove the tofu from the wok and set it aside.

5. Heat 2 more teaspoons of the oil in the wok over high heat. When the oil is hot, carefully add the bell pepper, zucchini, and bok choy to the wok. Cook the vegetables until they begin to soften, stirring often. Push the vegetables to one side of the wok and add the remaining teaspoon of oil to the bottom of the wok. Add the garlic and gingerroot to the oil and cook for 30 seconds. Stir all of the ingredients together.

6. Add the steamed wakami and broccoli to the wok. Add the tofu and remaining sauce to the wok. Cook the vegetables and tofu until hot, approximately 2 minutes, stirring often.

7. Transfer the stir-fry to a large platter and garnish with the soy nuts. Divide the rice among 4 plates and serve the meal family-style.

Bok Choy

Calcium-rich bok choy is an Asian cabbage with crunchy white stems and deep green leaves. Like Swiss chard, the entire plant is edible, but it's the crisp sweetness of the stem that makes this vegetable a standout on its own or as an ingredient in soups and stir-fries.

Choose small heads of bok choy over larger ones. Each stem of a small head can be sliced vertically, leaving the leaves intact. The stems of larger heads will need to be sliced horizontally into ¾-inch pieces and the leaves coarsely chopped.

Tempeh and Vegetable Burritos

Nutty-flavored tempeh and a splash of balsamic vinegar give these burritos unique flavor and texture. They contain a double dose of phytoestrogens from the tempeh and the soybeans used in the filling. Tips: *The soybean spread can be prepared up to 3 days in advance and refrigerated. Also, if a well-seasoned wok is used, no oil is necessary in step 5. If your wok is newer, a tablespoon of oil will be needed to prevent the vegetables from sticking.*

Preparation: 50 minutes
Cooking: 10 minutes
Yield: 4 main-course servings

BEANS

1 cup dried tomatoes
1 cup boiling water
2 15-ounce cans soybeans, drained and rinsed
1 small clove of garlic, peeled and crushed
Sea salt to taste
Black pepper to taste

REMAINING INGREDIENTS

3½ cups water
1½ cups short-grain brown rice
2 tablespoons canola oil, divided
8 ounces tempeh, cut into small cubes
2 tablespoons balsamic vinegar
2 Italian or Japanese eggplants, cubed
1 zucchini, cubed
1 red bell pepper, seeded and sliced
4 cloves garlic, peeled and sliced
4 ounces soy cheddar, grated or sliced
8 flour tortillas

1. Place the dried tomatoes in a bowl. Pour the boiling water on them. Allow to soften for 10 minutes or until soft. Drain and set aside.

2. Place the soybeans, rehydrated tomatoes, and garlic in the work bowl of a food processor that is fitted with a metal

blade. Puree the mixture until smooth, adding a small amount of water if necessary. Transfer to a bowl and season with sea salt and black pepper. Set the beans aside.

3. Meanwhile, bring the 3½ cups of water to a boil in a saucepan. Add the rice to the pan and return the water to a boil. Reduce the heat to a low simmer. Cover the pan and cook the rice until the water is absorbed, approximately 50 minutes. Set aside.

4. Toward the end of the rice cooking, heat 1 tablespoon of the oil in a well-seasoned wok over high heat. When the oil is hot, add the tempeh to the wok. Sear until golden, tossing 3 or 4 times. Remove the wok from the heat and drizzle the tempeh with the balsamic vinegar. Stir the tempeh and transfer to a plate.

5. Return the wok to high heat. When it is hot, add the eggplants, zucchini, and bell pepper. Cook the vegetables until they begin to soften, stirring 3 or 4 times.

6. Push the vegetables to one side of the wok and reduce the heat to medium. Add the remaining oil to the wok. Add the garlic cloves to the oil and cook for 30 seconds. Stir the garlic and vegetables together. Add the tempeh to the wok and stir thoroughly. Season the vegetables with sea salt and black pepper and transfer them to a large platter.

7. Melt a portion of soy cheddar on each flour tortilla (a microwave or slow oven works well). Spread a portion of the beans and rice on each tortilla. Place the platter of tempeh and vegetables on the table and have everyone fill and roll their own burritos.

Tofu, Corn, and Bell Pepper Fajitas with Spicy Soybeans

Preparation: 20 minutes
Cooking: 30 minutes
Yield: 4 main-course

Soybeans are a rich source of phytoestrogens, but they are not often used in cooking. This recipe combines soybeans and tofu, for a double phytoestrogen punch, with delicious vegetables, making a fajita the whole family will love. Tip: *The beans can be prepared a day in advance and refrigerated. Heat them in a microwave, stirring several times, before serving.*

BEANS

2 teaspoons olive oil

4 cloves garlic, peeled and sliced

1 medium onion, diced

½ Scotch bonnet pepper, seeded and chopped

4 scallions, trimmed and sliced, white and green parts separated

1 teaspoon chili powder

1 teaspoon cumin

½ teaspoon coriander

1 15-ounce can soybeans, drained and rinsed

½ cup cilantro, chopped

Sea salt to taste

Black pepper to taste

FAJITAS

2 tablespoons canola oil, divided

12 ounces firm tofu, sliced into small cubes

1 teaspoon chili powder, divided

1 teaspoon cumin, divided

1 teaspoon coriander, divided

4 ounces Jack cheese, grated or sliced

8 large flour tortillas

2 red bell peppers, seeded and sliced

1 large red onion, sliced

4 cloves garlic, peeled and thinly sliced

3 ears fresh corn, kernels removed, or 1½ cups frozen corn

Sea salt to taste

Black pepper to taste

1. To prepare the beans, heat the olive oil in a large skillet over low heat. Add the garlic to the skillet and cook until soft and fragrant. Add the onion, Scotch bonnet pepper, and the white parts of the scallions to the pan. Cook the ingredients until the

onion is soft, stirring often. Add the chili powder, cumin, and coriander and cook the ingredients 2 minutes longer.

2. Add the soybeans to the vegetables and cook together for two minutes.

3. Transfer the mixture to the work bowl of a food processor fitted with a metal blade and puree the mixture. Stir in the cilantro and the green parts of the scallions. Season the beans with sea salt and black pepper. Set aside.

4. To prepare the fajitas, heat the oven to 250°F. Heat one tablespoon of the oil in a well-seasoned wok over high heat. When the oil is hot, carefully add the tofu. Sear until golden, stirring 3 or 4 times. Add ½ teaspoon each of the chili powder, cumin, and coriander to the wok. Cook the tofu for 30 seconds longer. Remove from the pan and set aside.

5. Sprinkle an equal amount of the cheese on the tortillas. Place in the oven. Heat until the cheese melts and turn off the oven.

6. While the cheese is melting on the tortillas, heat the remaining tablespoon of oil in the wok over high heat. When it is hot, carefully add the bell peppers. Cook the peppers for one minute, stirring often. Add the onion to the wok and cook for two minutes. Continue stirring the vegetables. Add the garlic to the wok and cook for 30 seconds. Add the corn to the wok. Add the remaining dried spices and cook the ingredients for a final 30 seconds.

7. Return the tofu to the wok and stir all of the ingredients together. Season with sea salt and black pepper. Transfer the filling to a large platter.

8. Place the tortillas, filling, and beans on the table and allow people to fill and roll their own fajitas.

Tofu and Broccoli in Oyster Sauce

Preparation: 30 minutes
Cooking: 25 minutes
Yield: 4 main-course

Tofu and broccoli are a traditional Asian specialty and an excellent combination. The tofu takes on the flavor of the broccoli, and the oyster sauce flavors both. The tofu is a rich source of phytoestrogens, and the broccoli and bok choy are excellent sources of cal-

cium. Tip: *The broccoli can be steamed and the sauce prepared a day in advance.*

SAUCE
1 cup low-sodium chicken broth

2 tablespoons cider vinegar

4 tablespoons oyster sauce

3 tablespoons shoyu

1 teaspoon sugar

REMAINING INGREDIENTS
5 cups water, divided

2 cups sushi rice

Sea salt to taste

1 pound broccoli, trimmed, stems trimmed and cut into matchsticks, florets cut into 2-inch pieces

2 tablespoons canola oil, divided

1 pound firm tofu, sliced into small cubes

1 1-inch piece gingerroot, peeled and minced

3 cloves garlic, peeled and sliced

1 red bell pepper, cored and thinly sliced

8 ounces bok choy, trimmed, stems sliced diagonally into ¾-inch thick pieces and leaves coarsely chopped and separated

1. To prepare the sauce, whisk together the chicken broth, cider vinegar, oyster sauce, shoyu, and sugar in a bowl.

2. To complete the recipe, bring 4 cups of the water to a boil in a saucepan. Stir in the rice and bring the water back to a boil. Cover the pot, reduce the heat, and simmer the rice until it is tender and all of the water has been absorbed, approximately 25 minutes. Cover the rice and set aside.

3. While the rice is cooking, place the remaining cup of water in a Dutch oven and bring to a boil. Add a dash of sea salt to the water. Add the broccoli to the water, cover the pot, and steam for 5 minutes. Drain the broccoli and cool under running water. Set aside.

4. Heat 1 tablespoon of the oil in a wok over high heat.

When the oil is hot, add the tofu to the wok. Cook for 5 minutes, stirring occasionally. Transfer to a plate.

5. Heat the remaining tablespoon of oil in the wok over high heat. When the oil is hot, add the gingerroot and garlic to the wok and cook for 30 seconds. Add the bell pepper and bok choy stems to the wok. Cook until they begin to soften, stirring often. Add the bok choy leaves to the wok and cook for 30 seconds, stirring constantly.

6. Add the broccoli and tofu to the wok. Whisk the sauce and pour it into the wok. Cook the ingredients until hot, approximately 2 minutes, stirring occasionally. Transfer the meal to a large platter.

7. Divide the rice among 4 plates and serve family-style.

Chapter 16

Chicken and Pork Dishes

The health benefits gained from eating chicken are well documented. A skinless chicken breast is a lean protein source that is rich in niacin, riboflavin, and iron. Although a skinless chicken thigh contains slightly more fat than a breast, it is leaner than every cut of beef except the top round.

Pork finally is beginning to be known as a nutritious food. The fat content of well-trimmed pork loin is comparable to that of a skinless chicken thigh. The confusion in the past has been that pork is available in not only lean cuts but also very fatty cuts, such as spare ribs, bacon, and ham. Pork is a good source of iron, thiamin, and niacin.

The challenge in cooking with lean chicken breast and pork

loin is that the absence of fat can be accompanied by an absence of flavor. However, a skinless chicken breast or a thin slice of pork loin is to a cook what a canvas is to an artist—something plain that with creativity can be transformed into something wonderful. The mild taste of chicken breast and pork loin stand up well to robust flavors such as lemon, wine, mustard, balsamic vinegar, and blue cheese. How do you combine those flavors without using an inordinate amount of butter, oil, or cream?

Combining chicken and pork with soy can be a creative answer to that problem. Initially, we thought the only way to pair soy with anything other than vegetables was the Asian favorite, Tofu and Beef in Oyster Sauce. We take you beyond this ubiquitous dish and offer other intriguing possibilities pairing chicken or pork with soy. Silken tofu can be pureed and added to intensely flavored, broth-based liquids to create delectable sauces.

A favorite restaurant meal of ours is mustard chicken, a skinless chicken breast slathered in a rich, creamy mustard sauce. Our version is just as flavorful and just as creamy with silken tofu replacing the cream. The quickly prepared dish of Pan-Seared Pork Loin with Shallots and Red Wine is another winner—tender slices of pork topped with a rich, full-bodied wine and tofu sauce. We also offer a version of a traditional favorite, Chicken Ragu—slow-cooked skinless chicken thighs in a tomato-cream sauce. Instead of finishing the sauce with cream, we finish it with silken tofu. When silken tofu is used to bind and enrich a sauce, it is possible to enjoy rich-tasting, low-fat, and phytoestrogen-rich chicken and pork meals.

Two-Mustard Chicken

Preparation: 10 minutes
Cooking: 15 minutes
Yield: 4 main-course servings

Do not be fooled by the creaminess of this phytoestrogen-rich mustard sauce. It is satiny because of the addition of heart-healthy silken tofu, not heavy cream, making this dish a perfect way to serve boneless chicken breasts for a healthy menopause diet. Tip:

When adding the mustard sauce to the pan, do so over low heat to prevent the sauce from curdling.

6 ounces silken tofu

1 tablespoon Dijon mustard

2 tablespoons whole-seed mustard

Sea salt to taste

Black pepper to taste

3 teaspoons canola oil, divided

1½ pounds boneless and skinless chicken breast, cut into 4 pieces and flattened to 1/4-inch thickness

3 medium shallots, peeled and chopped

12 ounces white mushrooms, sliced

12 ounces low-sodium chicken broth

1. Place the tofu and mustards in the work bowl of a food processor fitted with a metal blade and process until smooth. Season with sea salt and black pepper.

2. Heat 1 teaspoon of the oil in a large skillet over high heat. Sprinkle the chicken pieces on each side with sea salt and black pepper. When the oil is hot, carefully place the chicken in the skillet. Sear the chicken pieces on each side. Transfer to a plate.

3. Reduce the heat to low and add the remaining 2 teaspoons of oil to the skillet. Add the shallots and cook until soft, stirring often.

4. Raise the heat to medium and add the mushrooms to the skillet. Sprinkle with sea salt and cook until soft.

5. Raise the heat to high, add the broth to the skillet and bring to a boil. Simmer for 5 minutes.

6. Return the chicken pieces to the pan. Reduce the heat and simmer for 2 minutes.

7. Divide the chicken among 4 plates. Remove the skillet from the heat and stir in the mustard sauce. Spoon a portion of the sauce onto each serving. Accompany with Monique's New Potatoes with Cucumber Raita (see page 280).

Chicken with Cilantro and Scallions

Preparation: 10 minutes
Cooking: 15 minutes
Yield: 4 main-course servings

Boneless chicken breasts are quick, easy, and low in fat and calories. Their neutral flavor makes them the ideal canvas for an intensely flavored sauce. Silken tofu makes this simple, yet flavorful sauce rich in phytoestrogens.

2 plum tomatoes, diced
4 Kalamata olives, pitted and chopped
1 tablespoon chili powder
2 teaspoons ground cumin
1 teaspoon dried coriander
1 teaspoon oregano
½ teaspoon cayenne
1 cup fresh cilantro, chopped
3 scallions, trimmed and sliced
3 tablespoons slivered almonds
6 ounces silken tofu
Sea salt to taste
Black pepper to taste
3 teaspoons canola oil, divided
1½ pounds boneless and skinless chicken breasts, cut into 4 pieces and flattened to 1/4-inch thickness
3 cloves garlic, peeled and sliced
12 ounces low-sodium chicken broth

1. In a small bowl combine the tomatoes and olives and set aside for a garnish.

2. In another bowl create the spice mixture by combining the chili powder, cumin, dried coriander, oregano, and cayenne.

3. Place the cilantro, scallions, and almonds in the work bowl of a food processor fitted with a metal blade. Process the ingredients until well combined. Add the tofu to the work bowl and process the ingredients until smooth. Season the sauce with sea salt and black pepper. Transfer to a bowl and set aside.

4. Heat 2 teaspoons of the oil in a large skillet over high

heat. Sprinkle the chicken pieces on each side with the spice mixture. When the oil is hot, carefully place the chicken in the skillet. Cook the chicken pieces on both sides until done. Transfer the chicken to a plate.

5. Reduce the heat to low and add the remaining teaspoon of oil to the pan. Add the garlic to the pan and cook until soft and fragrant.

6. Raise the heat to high and add the broth to the skillet. Bring the broth to a boil and simmer for 5 minutes.

7. Divide the chicken among 4 plates. Remove the pan from the heat and stir in the cilantro-scallion sauce. Spoon a portion of the sauce onto each serving and garnish with the tomatoes and olives. Accompany with Spicy Brown Rice (see page 283).

Chicken Ragu

In Italian cooking ragu refers to a slow-cooked meat sauce that is finished with cream and often accompanied with polenta or pasta. We have prepared this version using chicken and pureed silken tofu, which makes it much lower in fat and calories and rich in phytoestrogens.

Preparation: 20 minutes
Cooking: 2 hours
Yield: 6 main-course servings

1 tablespoon olive oil
8 bone-in, skinless chicken thighs, rinsed and dried
Sea salt to taste
Black pepper to taste
6 cloves garlic, peeled and sliced
1 large onion, peeled and diced
1 carrot, peeled and diced
2 ribs celery, diced
1½ cups dry red wine
2 28-ounce cans whole tomatoes, chopped
½ cup flat-leaf parsley, chopped
6 ounces silken tofu, pureed

1. Heat the oven to 275°F. Heat the olive oil in a large Dutch oven over high heat. Sprinkle the chicken thighs with sea salt and pepper and carefully place them in the oil. Sear the thighs on each side, turning them once. Remove the thighs from the pot and reduce the heat to low.

2. Add the garlic to the pot and cook until soft and fragrant. Add the onion to the pot and cook until soft, stirring occasionally. Raise the heat slightly, add the carrot and celery to the pot, and sprinkle with sea salt. Cover the pot and steam for 5 minutes.

3. Return the thighs to the pot along with any accumulated juices. Cover the pot and steam the ingredients for 10 minutes. Raise the heat to high, add the wine to the pot, and simmer for 3 minutes.

4. Add the tomatoes to the pot and bring the sauce to a boil. Cover the pot and place in the oven. Braise the chicken thighs for 1¼ hours.

5. Remove the pot from the oven and return to the stove. Uncover the pot and reduce the sauce over medium heat for 15 minutes, stirring occasionally.

6. Stir the parsley into the sauce. Season with sea salt and black pepper.

7. Remove the chicken from the pot and place on a platter. Stir the tofu into the sauce. Transfer the sauce to a serving bowl. Serve the meal family style and accompany with Polenta (see page 272).

Lemon–Ginger Chicken and Tofu

Preparation: 20 minutes
Cooking: 25 minutes
Yield: 4 main-course servings

Tofu is not just for vegetarians. It is often used in Asian cooking combined with beef, chicken, or fish. In this dish phytoestrogen-rich tofu is combined with a lemon-ginger chicken, a combination that is refreshing and delicious.

Lemon Sauce

Juice from 2 lemons

1 cup low-sodium canned chicken broth

1 tablespoon sesame oil

1 tablespoon sugar

Remaining Ingredients

4 cups water, divided

1½ cups sushi rice

Sea salt to taste

1 bunch broccoli, trimmed and sliced into large florets

½ pound asparagus, tough part of stems snapped off and discarded, stalks loosely tied together

Vegetable steaming water

2 tablespoons canola oil, divided

12 ounces boneless, skinless chicken breast, thinly sliced

12 ounces firm tofu, cut into small cubes

1 1-inch piece gingerroot, peeled and minced

2 red bell peppers, cored and julienned

Black pepper to taste

½ cup fresh cilantro, chopped

1. To prepare the sauce, whisk together lemon juice, chicken broth, sesame oil, and sugar. Set aside.

2. To complete the recipe, bring 3 cups of the water to a boil in a saucepan. Stir the rice into the water. Cover the pot, reduce the heat, and simmer until all of the water has been absorbed, approximately 20 minutes. Set aside.

3. While the rice is cooking, bring the remaining cup of water to a boil in a Dutch oven and add a dash of sea salt. Add the broccoli and asparagus to the water. Cover the pot and steam for 6 minutes. Drain the vegetables and reserve their water. Run the vegetables under cold water to stop the cooking process. Stir their steaming water into the sauce.

4. Heat 1 tablespoon of the canola oil in a wok over high heat. When the oil is hot, carefully place the chicken and tofu into the wok. Sear the ingredients, stirring 3 or 4 times. Whisk

the sauce and add 4 tablespoons of it to the chicken and tofu. Cook until the sauce is absorbed. Transfer the ingredients to a plate and set aside.

5. Heat the remaining tablespoon of oil in the wok over high heat. Add the gingerroot to the oil and cook for 30 seconds. Add bell peppers and cook until they begin to soften.

6. Add the vegetables, chicken, and tofu to the wok. Whisk the remaining sauce and add it to the wok. Cook the ingredients until they are hot. Season with sea salt and black pepper. Remove the wok from the heat and stir in the cilantro. Transfer the stir-fry to a large platter.

7. Divide the rice among 4 plates and serve the meal family-style.

Curried Chicken and Bok Choy

Preparation: 15 minutes
Cooking: 15 minutes
Yield: 4 main-course servings

This chicken dish is served with a curry-tofu sauce that is rich in phytoestrogens. The silken tofu takes on the curry flavor, while adding a richness to the sauce. The stir-fried bok choy adds contrasting color and texture, as well as additional calcium. Tip: *The curry-tofu sauce can be prepared a day in advance and refrigerated. Also, when adding the curry-tofu sauce to the pan, do so over low heat to prevent the sauce from curdling.*

5 teaspoons canola oil, divided
3 cloves garlic, peeled and sliced
1 1-inch piece gingerroot, peeled and sliced
1 onion, peeled and diced
2 tablespoons curry powder, divided
3 tablespoons water
8 ounces silken tofu
Sea salt to taste
Black pepper to taste
1 pound boneless and skinless chicken breast, thinly sliced
8 ounces bok choy, trimmed, stems sliced diagonally into

¾-inch thick pieces and leaves coarsely chopped
1 cup low-sodium chicken broth

1. Heat 2 teaspoons of the oil in a skillet over low heat. Add the garlic and ginger to the pan and cook until soft and fragrant. Add the onion to the pan and cook it until soft.

2. Add 1 tablespoon of the curry powder to the skillet and cook the ingredients for 2 minutes longer, stirring often. Add the water to the skillet and remove from the heat.

3. Transfer ingredients to the work bowl of a food processor fitted with a metal blade. Process ingredients until smooth. Add tofu to the work bowl and process ingredients until a smooth sauce forms. Season with sea salt and black pepper and set aside.

4. Heat 2 more teaspoons of the oil in the skillet over high heat. Toss the chicken with the sea salt, black pepper, and the remaining tablespoon of curry powder. When the oil is hot, add the chicken breast to the skillet. Cook the chicken until golden, stirring occasionally. Transfer to a plate.

5. Heat the remaining teaspoon of oil in the pan over high heat. When it is hot, add the bok choy. Cook the bok choy for three minutes, stirring often.

6. Add the chicken broth to the skillet and bring to a boil. Reduce the heat and simmer the bok choy until tender.

7. Return the chicken to the skillet. Stir the curry-tofu sauce into the skillet. Season with sea salt and black pepper.

8. Divide the chicken among 4 plates and accompany with Basmati Rice with Almonds and Raisins (see page 249).

Chicken with Tempeh, White Beans, Tomatoes, and Basil

The combination of chicken and beans is a traditional Tuscan specialty. We add tempeh to the sauce to absorb some of the wonderful flavors in this dish and to add a dose of phytoestrogens. The

Preparation: 20 minutes
Cooking: 1½ hours
Yield: 6 main-course servings

beans add fiber that otherwise would be lacking in this dish. Tip:
To save time during cleanup, use the cover as a plate for the
chicken after it has been seared. Any chicken juices that have
accumulated on the cover should be added to the sauce.

1 tablespoon olive oil

8 skinless chicken thighs, rinsed and dried

Sea salt to taste

Black pepper to taste

6 cloves garlic, divided, peeled, and sliced

1 onion, peeled and diced

1 stalk celery, diced

1 carrot, peeled and diced

1 cup white wine

1 15-ounce can low-sodium chicken broth

1 28-ounce can whole tomatoes, chopped

12 ounces tempeh, cubed

1 15-ounce can Great Northern or navy beans, drained and
  rinsed

½ cup fresh basil

1. Heat the olive oil in a large Dutch oven over high heat.
Sprinkle the chicken thighs on each side with sea salt and
black pepper. Carefully place them in the hot oil and sear each
on both sides, turning once. Remove the chicken from the pot
and set aside.

2. Reduce the heat to low and add 4 cloves of garlic to the
pot. Cook the garlic until soft and fragrant, stirring constantly.
Add the onion to the pot and cook until it begins to soften,
stirring often.

3. Add the celery, carrot, and a pinch of sea salt to the pot.
Cover the pot and steam for 5 minutes, stirring occasionally.

4. Raise the heat to high and add the wine to the pot and
simmer for two minutes. Add the broth, tomatoes, tempeh,
and seared chicken thighs to the pot. Bring the sauce to a boil
and then reduce the heat to a low simmer. Cover the pot and
cook the stew for 1 hour, stirring occasionally.

5. Add the beans to the stew and raise the heat to medium. Cook the stew, uncovered, for 15 minutes, stirring occasionally.

6. Season the stew with sea salt and black pepper. Thoroughly chop the basil and remaining garlic together and stir into the sauce.

7. Accompany the stew with Polenta (see page 272).

Chicken with Arugula Pesto and Dried Tomatoes

This dish was created using fresh arugula from our garden. Arugula makes an intensely flavored pesto, and our version is made with silken tofu instead of olive oil, so it is low in fat yet rich in phytoestrogens. Tips: *When adding the pesto sauce to the pan, do so over low heat to prevent the sauce from curdling. The pesto can be prepared a day in advance and refrigerated.*

Preparation: 15 minutes
Cooking: 15 minutes
Yield: 4 main-course servings

1 cup dried tomatoes
1 cup boiling water
1 bunch arugula (2 cups), trimmed, washed, and drained
½ cup fresh basil
1 small clove garlic, peeled and minced
¼ cup pine nuts
¼ cup grated Parmesan cheese
6 ounces silken tofu
Sea salt to taste
Black pepper to taste
3 teaspoons canola oil, divided
1½ pounds boneless and skinless chicken breast, cut into 4
    pieces and flattened to 1/4-inch thickness
2 medium shallots, peeled and chopped
12 ounces low-sodium chicken broth

1. Place the dried tomatoes in a bowl and pour the boiling water on them. Allow to macerate for 10 minutes or until soft. Drain and coarsely chop the tomatoes. Set aside.

2. Place the arugula, basil, garlic, pine nuts, and Parmesan cheese in the work bowl of a food processor fitted with a metal blade. Process the ingredients until they are well combined. Add the tofu and process until smooth. Season with sea salt and black pepper. Transfer the pesto sauce to a bowl and set aside.

3. Heat 1 teaspoon of the oil in a large skillet over high heat. Sprinkle the chicken pieces on each side with sea salt and black pepper. When the oil is hot, carefully place the chicken pieces in the skillet. Sear on each side, turning once. Transfer to a plate.

4. Reduce the heat to low and add the remaining 2 teaspoons of oil to the skillet. Add the shallots and cook until soft, stirring often.

5. Raise the heat to high and add the broth and tomatoes to the skillet. Bring the broth to a boil. Return the chicken pieces to the pan. Reduce the heat and simmer for 2 minutes.

6. Divide the chicken among 4 plates. Remove the skillet from the heat and stir in the pesto sauce. Spoon a portion of the sauce onto each serving. Accompany with Elbow Macaroni Salad (see page 284).

Pan–Seared Pork Loin with Shallots and Red Wine

Preparation: 10 minutes
Cooking: 15 minutes
Yield: 4 main-course servings

With few ingredients and a short preparation time, this is a low-fat and heart-healthy meal you can enjoy on a regular basis. Silken tofu adds richness and texture to the sauce. Tip: *To achieve great flavor in this dish without the use of a rich stock, it is important to sear the pork. The searing will ensure that the sauce is flavorful from the caramelized bits, which will dissolve when you deglaze the pan (see step 5).*

6 ounces silken tofu

2 teaspoons canola oil, divided

1 pound pork loin, cut into 4 medallions

Sea salt to taste

Black pepper to taste

2 medium shallots, peeled and finely chopped

⅔ cup dry red wine

⅔ cup low-sodium canned chicken broth

1. Place the tofu in a food processor fitted with a metal blade and puree it. Set aside.

2. Heat 1 teaspoon of the oil in a cast-iron skillet over high heat. Pat the pork medallions dry and sprinkle on each side with sea salt and black pepper.

3. When the oil is hot, carefully place the pork medallions in the skillet. Sear on each side, turning once. Remove the medallions from the pan and set aside.

4. Reduce the heat to low and add the remaining teaspoon of oil to the pan. Add the shallots to the pan and cook until soft, stirring constantly.

5. Raise the heat to high and add the wine to the skillet. With a spoon, scrape the skillet to dissolve the caramelized bits. Add the chicken broth to the pan and reduce the sauce for 3 minutes. Reduce the heat to low and stir in the tofu.

6. Return the pork to the pan and cook for 3 more minutes, turning occasionally.

7. Divide the pork among 4 plates. Season the sauce with sea salt and black pepper. Spoon the sauce onto the pork. Accompany with Israeli Couscous with Broccoli Rabe and Raisins (see page 278).

Pork Loin with Dried Tomatoes, Artichoke Hearts, and Olives

Preparation: 20 minutes
Cooking: 15 minutes
Yield: 4 main-course servings

This is one of our favorite pork recipes, a delicious medley of flavors and ingredients. Serve it with Garlic Mashed Potatoes (see page 273) for a perfect low-fat and phytoestrogen-rich accompaniment.

½ cup dried tomatoes
1 cup boiling water
2 teaspoons canola oil, divided
1 pound pork loin, cut into 4 medallions
Sea salt to taste
Black pepper to taste
1 shallot, peeled and finely chopped
½ cup dry white wine
1 cup low-sodium canned chicken broth
1 tablespoon unsalted butter (optional)
4 canned artichoke hearts, quartered
10 Kalamata olives, pitted and chopped

1. Place the dried tomatoes in a bowl and pour the boiling water on them. Allow to macerate for 10 minutes or until soft. Drain and coarsely chop the tomatoes. Set aside.

2. Heat 1 teaspoon of the oil in a cast-iron skillet over high heat. Pat the pork medallions dry and sprinkle on each side with sea salt and black pepper.

3. When the oil is hot, carefully place the pork medallions in the skillet. Sear on each side, turning once. Remove the medallions and set aside.

4. Reduce the heat to low and add the remaining teaspoon of oil to the skillet. Add the shallot and cook until soft, stirring constantly.

5. Raise the heat to high and add the wine to the skillet. With a spoon scrape the skillet to dissolve the caramelized bits. Add the chicken broth. If desired, add the butter at this time.

6. Return the pork to the skillet and cook for 3 more minutes, turning occasionally.

7. Divide the pork among 4 plates. Raise the heat to high under the sauce and add the artichoke hearts, olives, and tomatoes. Cook the sauce for 2 more minutes. Season with sea salt and black pepper. Spoon the sauce onto the pork and serve at once.

Pork with Capers and Lemon

The pork loin is the leanest cut, almost as lean as skinless chicken breast. Pork therefore can be part of a heart-healthy diet if prepared correctly. This very quick and simple preparation is delicious served with Fettuccine with a Tomato "Cream" Sauce (see page 191), which is a phytoestrogen-rich and low-fat dish. Tip: This recipe also works well with boneless and skinless chicken breasts.

Preparation: 10 minutes
Cooking: 15 minutes
Yield: 4 main-course servings

3 teaspoons olive oil, divided
1 pound pork loin, cut into 4 medallions
Sea salt to taste
Black pepper to taste
2 cloves garlic, peeled and sliced
2 shallots, peeled and finely chopped
1 cup dry white wine
1 cup low-sodium chicken broth
Juice from 1 lemon
2 tablespoons capers, drained and rinsed
4 tablespoons flat-leaf parsley, chopped

1. Heat 1 teaspoon of the olive oil in a skillet over high heat. Sprinkle the pork on each side with sea salt and black pepper. When the oil is hot, place the pork in the skillet.

2. Sear the pork on each side, turning once. Transfer the pork to a plate and set aside.

3. Add the remaining 2 teaspoons of oil to the skillet and reduce the heat to low. Add the garlic and cook for 30 seconds. Add the shallots and cook until soft, stirring constantly.

4. Raise the heat to high, add the wine to the skillet, and simmer for 2 minutes. Add the broth and bring to a boil. Return the pork to the skillet.

5. Reduce the heat and simmer the sauce and pork for 5 minutes, turning the pork occasionally.

6. Divide the pork among 4 plates. Raise the heat to high and reduce the sauce for 2 minutes.

7. Remove the skillet from the heat and add the lemon, capers, and parsley. Season the sauce with sea salt and black pepper. Spoon the sauce onto the pork and serve at once.

Jambalaya

Preparation: 20 minutes
Cooking: 1½ hours
Yield: 6 main-course servings

Jambalaya is a Creole dish traditionally made with a pork-based andouille sausage. Here we have substituted andouille sausage made with turkey, which is much leaner than the pork variety. We also have added tofu, which absorbs the wonderful flavors from the variety of ingredients and adds a healthy dose of phytoestrogens. Tips: *If you can't find turkey andouille sausage, use a spicy Italian turkey or chicken sausage. Also, the broth base can be prepared earlier in the day. An hour before serving, bring the broth to a boil and add the rice and proceed with the recipe.*

2 dried chili peppers
2 cups boiling water
2 teaspoons canola oil
6 bone-in, skinless chicken thighs, rinsed and dried
Sea salt to taste
8 ounces turkey andouille sausage, sliced
6 cloves garlic, peeled and sliced
1 onion, peeled and diced
1 green bell pepper, seeded and sliced

1 red bell pepper, seeded and sliced
1 tablespoon chili powder
Reserved chili pepper–soaking water
1 28-ounce can whole tomatoes, chopped
1 pound firm tofu, rinsed and sliced into small cubes
Black pepper to taste
2 cups short-grain brown rice

1. Place the chili peppers in a bowl and pour the water on them. Allow to soften for 15 minutes. Remove from the water and reserve the water for the broth. Seed and chop them. Set aside.

2. While the peppers are soaking, heat the oil in a Dutch oven over high heat. Sprinkle the chicken thighs with sea salt and carefully place them in the hot oil. Scatter the sausage slices around the chicken. Sear the chicken until a crust forms, turning once. Remove the chicken and sausage from the pot and set aside.

3. Reduce the heat to low and add the garlic to the pot. Cook the garlic until soft and fragrant. Add the onion to the pot and cook until soft, stirring occasionally.

4. Add the green and red peppers and chili powder to the pot and sprinkle the ingredients with sea salt. Cover the pot and steam the vegetables for 5 minutes, stirring occasionally. Return the chicken and sausage to the pot and steam for 10 minutes longer.

5. Add the softened chilies and their soaking water to the pot. Bring the liquid to a boil, reduce the heat, cover the pot, and simmer for 5 minutes.

6. Add the tomatoes and tofu to the pot and bring the liquid to a boil. Reduce the heat, cover the pot, and simmer the broth for 15 minutes. Season with sea salt and black pepper.

7. Return the broth to a boil and stir in the rice. Reduce the heat, cover the pot, and simmer the rice until it is tender, approximately 45 minutes.

8. Divide the Jambalaya among 6 plates and accompany with rustic bread.

Chapter 17

Seafood Dishes

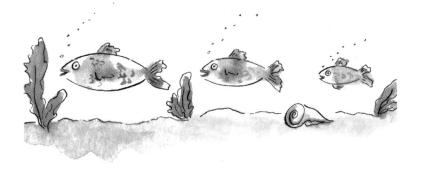

At first glance fish and soy may seem like an odd combination, but they actually work quite well together. By combining fish and soy, you can enhance the wonderful nutrition seafood offers. At the same time you will be creating wonderful meals that are rich in flavor and phytoestrogens.

The nutritional profile of most of the fish available in today's markets is amazing. Lean fish, such as cod, haddock, and flounder, and shellfish, such as mussels, clams, and shrimp, are all very low in saturated fat. Even fish that are considered fatty, like salmon, bluefish, and swordfish, are rich in omega-3 fatty acids, important in the prevention of heart disease. Seafood is also a wonderfully lean protein source. It is comparable to skinless chicken breast. In addition, oysters, mussels, and clams are a good source of iron. Canned salmon is an excellent source of calcium. When you combine all of this wonderful seafood nutrition with soy, you create delicious menopausal meals.

Indulge in Pan-Seared Salmon with Creamed Spinach and Lemon. You can tell your family and friends to relax and enjoy their meal since the creamy texture of the spinach is from pureed silken tofu. Or try the Roasted Cod with a White Bean and Dried-Tomato Ragu. Again, the flavor and texture of this hearty dish are enhanced with silken tofu. If you are craving a fish stew, try our hearty spicy Portuguese Fish Stew. For a double dose of phytoestrogens, accompany it with Soy Polenta to soak up the wonderful juices.

As you can see from these recipes, it is possible to combine soy and seafood creatively and turn them into delectable meals and phytoestrogen powerhouses. So yes, it is possible to have your seafood and eat your soy, too.

Shrimp with Dried Tomatoes, Tofu, Basil, and Balsamic Vinegar

We use fresh Maine shrimp in this recipe when they are in season. If you can locate them, they are a real treat. Frozen shrimp are widely available and are a fine substitute. Although higher in cholesterol than other fish, shrimp are overall still low in fat and calories. Quickly cooking the shrimp in a vinegar-based sauce is a simple and low-fat cooking method. Tofu is a wonderful addition, since it will absorb the flavors of the shrimp, vinegar, and basil. Tips: *Squid or sea scallops can be substituted for the shrimp. Also, the dried tomatoes can be softened a day in advance. Store both the tomatoes and their soaking water, covered, in the refrigerator.*

Preparation: 10 minutes
Cooking: 10 minutes
Yield: 6 main-course servings

1 cup dried tomatoes
1 cup boiling water
2 tablespoons olive oil, divided
8 ounces firm tofu, cut into small cubes
5 tablespoons top-quality balsamic vinegar, divided
5 cloves garlic, peeled and thinly sliced
Tomato-soaking water
1½ pounds large shrimp, peeled and deveined
½ cup fresh basil, snipped
Sea salt to taste
Black pepper to taste

1. Place the dried tomatoes in a bowl and pour the water on them. Allow to macerate for 10 minutes or until soft. Drain and reserve soaking water. Coarsely chop and set aside.

2. Heat 1 tablespoon of the olive oil in a wok over high heat. When the oil is hot, add the tofu and cook until it is golden, stirring occasionally. Add 3 tablespoons of the vinegar to the wok and cook the tofu for 30 seconds more. Transfer to a plate and set aside.

3. Heat the remaining tablespoon of olive oil in the wok over high heat. When the oil is hot, add the garlic and cook for 30 seconds, stirring constantly. Add the tomato-soaking water to the wok and bring to a boil.

4. Put the shrimp, remaining 2 tablespoons of vinegar, and basil into the pot, stirring occasionally. Cook the ingredients until the shrimp turn pink. Stir in the tofu. Season with sea salt and black pepper.

5. Transfer the shrimp and tofu to a large platter and accompany with crusty bread.

Pan-Seared Salmon with Creamed Spinach and Lemon

Salmon is a fish rich in heart-healthy omega-3 fatty acids. You should try to eat such fatty fish often for a heart-healthy diet. The greens, made creamy with silken tofu, are a perfect visual and taste complement to the sweet fish. They also add healthful doses of phytoestrogens and antioxidants. Tip: *Swordfish or striped bass can be substituted for the salmon. Ask your fishmonger to skin the fish for you. A well-seasoned cast-iron skillet is the cooking vessel of choice in this recipe.*

Preparation: 10 minutes
Cooking: 10 minutes
Yield: 4-main course servings

1 tablespoon canola oil
1 pound salmon fillet, cut from the thick end, skinned and cut into 4 pieces
Sea salt to taste
Black pepper to taste
2 teaspoons olive oil
2 cloves garlic, peeled and sliced
1½ pounds fresh spinach, trimmed, chopped, washed, and drained
½ cup dry white wine
Juice from 1 lemon
6 ounces silken tofu, pureed
1 lemon, cut into 4 wedges

1. Heat the canola oil in a heavy skillet over high heat. Sprinkle the fish on each side with sea salt and black pepper. When the oil is hot, carefully place the fish in the skillet. Sear on each side, turning once. Reduce the heat and finish cooking the fish. Transfer to a warm plate.

2. Heat the olive oil in the skillet over high heat. When the oil is hot, add the garlic to the skillet and cook for 30 seconds. Stir the spinach into the pan. Pour the wine into the pan and cook the spinach until it wilts, stirring constantly.

Remove the skillet from the heat and stir in the lemon juice and tofu. Season the spinach with sea salt and black pepper.

3. Divide the spinach among 4 plates. Place a piece of salmon on each portion of spinach. Accompany with lemon wedges and Garlic Mashed Potatoes (see page 273).

Baked Cod with Tomatoes and Breadcrumbs

Preparation: 20 minutes
Cooking: 20 minutes
Yield: 4 main-course servings

Whitefish, such as cod, are low in fat, cholesterol, and calories and simple to prepare. Try to eat fish at least once a week. Silken tofu is pureed and added to the tomato-parsley sauce, making it creamy and phytoestrogen rich. Tips: *The tomato-parsley sauce can be prepared a day in advance and refrigerated. Monkfish, haddock, or hake can be substituted for the cod.*

TOMATO-PARSLEY SAUCE

1 tablespoon olive oil
4 cloves garlic, peeled and sliced
1 onion, peeled and diced
⅔ cup dry white wine
1 28-ounce can whole tomatoes, chopped
6 ounces silken tofu, pureed
⅓ cup flat-leaf parsley, chopped
Sea salt to taste
Black pepper to taste

REMAINING INGREDIENTS

1 pound cod fillet (preferably cut from the thick end), cut into 4 pieces
1 cup tomato-parsley sauce
⅔ cup dry white wine
2 cups fresh breadcrumbs (see page 275)
12 ounces penne

1. Heat the oven to 400°F. Bring a large pot of water to a boil.

2. To prepare the sauce, heat the olive oil in a Dutch oven over low heat. Add the garlic to the pot and cook until soft and fragrant. Add the onion to the pot and cook until soft, stirring occasionally.

3. Raise the heat to high and add the wine to the pot. Simmer for 2 minutes. Add the tomatoes and bring the sauce to a boil. Reduce the heat and simmer for 15 minutes, stirring occasionally.

4. Stir the tofu and parsley into the sauce. Season with sea salt and black pepper and set aside.

5. To prepare the fish, place it in an oven-proof casserole. Mix the cup of tomato-parsley sauce and wine together and pour it on the fish. Pack the breadcrumbs with your hands and place them on top of the fish.

6. Place the fish in the oven. Bake until the sauce just begins to bubble, approximately 12–15 minutes. Turn on the broiler and broil the fish until the breadcrumbs are golden.

7. After the fish has been cooking for 7 minutes, add sea salt to the boiling water followed by the pasta.

8. Remove the fish from the oven. Drain the pasta and toss with the remaining tomato-parsley sauce.

9. Divide the fish among 4 plates. Place a portion of pasta on each plate and serve immediately.

Portuguese Fish Stew

Chouriço is a Portuguese sausage, which gives this fish stew wonderful flavor. In this version we use a chicken chouriço, much lower in fat than the traditional pork variety. The remainder of the stew is based upon fish and shellfish, which, when combined with the smoky sausage, make a delectable combination. The unusual ingredient in the dish is silken tofu. It creates a smooth-tasting sauce that seems to cling to your palate. Tip: *The tomato-*

Preparation: 15 minutes
Cooking: 30 minutes
Yield: 4 main-course servings

chouriço sauce (without the tofu) can be prepared a day in advance and refrigerated.

1 tablespoon olive oil
6 ounces chicken chouriço or hot Italian chicken or turkey sausage, diced
6 cloves garlic, peeled and sliced
1 onion, peeled and diced
1½ cups dry white wine
42 ounces (1½ 28-ounce cans) whole tomatoes, chopped
1 pound thick-cut cod, cut into 4 pieces
2 pounds mussels, scrubbed and debearded
1 pound cleaned squid, bodies sliced into rounds and tentacles halved if large
1 pound medium or large shrimp, peeled and deveined
Sea salt to taste
Black pepper to taste
½ cup fresh basil, snipped
6 ounces silken tofu, pureed

1. Heat the olive oil in a Dutch oven over high heat. Add the chouriço to the pot and cook until well browned. Remove and set aside.

2. Reduce the heat to low. Add the garlic to the pot and cook until soft. Add the onion to the pot and cook until soft.

3. Raise the heat to high, add the wine to the pot, and simmer for 2 minutes. Add the tomatoes and bring the sauce to a boil. Reduce the heat and simmer for 20 minutes, stirring occasionally.

4. Raise the heat to high. When the sauce boils, add the cod to the pot and cook for 2 minutes.

5. Add the mussels to the pot and cook until they just begin to open.

6. Add the squid and shrimp to the pot and cook for 2 minutes. Remove the pot from the heat. Season the sauce with sea salt and black pepper. Stir in the basil and tofu.

7. Divide the stew among 4 large bowls. Accompany with rustic bread and Romaine Salad with Garlic Croutons and Lemon (see page 166).

Poached Salmon with Couscous and Vegetables

Poaching is a heart-healthy technique for preparing fish by gently simmering it in a skillet in broth. Here, omega-3 fatty acid–rich salmon is served with bok choy, a green that is rich in calcium and antioxidants. Tip: *Although it would seem more sensible to poach the fish in the broth for the couscous, we found the resulting liquid to be too strongly flavored. Poaching the fish in a separate pan is a better method. The poaching broth can be frozen and used later to flavor a soup or sauce.*

Preparation: 15 minutes
Cooking: 15 minutes
Yield: 4 main-course servings

COUSCOUS

2 cups Israeli couscous

Sea salt to taste

3 cups vegetable broth or water

1 carrot, peeled and sliced into matchsticks

1 leek, trimmed, washed, and sliced

4 ounces bok choy, trimmed, stems sliced into matchsticks, leaves chopped and kept separate

1 zucchini, sliced into matchsticks

½ cup fresh basil, snipped

Black pepper to taste

REMAINING INGREDIENTS

4 cups vegetable broth

1 tablespoon olive oil

Sea salt to taste

1½ pounds salmon fillet, preferably cut from the thick end, skinned

1. To prepare the couscous, bring a pot of water to a boil. Add sea salt to the water, followed by the couscous. Cook the couscous until it is tender, approximately 4 minutes. Drain and set aside.

2. Meanwhile, place the 3 cups of vegetable broth or water in a Dutch oven and bring to a boil. Reduce the heat and add the carrot to the pot. Simmer the carrot for 2 minutes. Add the leek and simmer for 2 minutes. Add the bok choy stems and zucchini. Simmer for 2 more minutes. Stir in the bok choy leaves and basil. Season the broth with sea salt and black pepper and set it aside.

3. To complete the recipe, bring the remaining 4 cups of vegetable broth to a boil in a skillet. Add the olive oil and a dash of sea salt. Reduce the heat to a low simmer (approximately 190°F).

4. Place the fish in the broth and cover the pan. Poach the fish until it is cooked through, approximately 10 minutes. Remove the skillet from the heat.

5. Stir the vegetable mixture into the couscous. Divide the couscous, broth, and vegetables among 4 shallow bowls. Place a portion of fish in each bowl and serve immediately.

Pan-Seared Tuna with Goat Cheese, Leeks, and Basil

Preparation: 10 minutes
Cooking: 15 minutes
Yield: 4 main-course servings

Tuna is a fish rich in omega-3 fatty acids, which fight artery-clogging plaques to prevent atherosclerotic heart disease. This is a simple pan-seared version that makes for a quick and easy preparation. Goat cheese is a relatively low-fat cheese that is a good source of calcium. Tip: *You can substitute salmon and swordfish for the tuna.*

4 teaspoons canola oil, divided
1¼ pounds tuna steaks, cut into 4 pieces
Sea salt to taste
Black pepper to taste
4 ounces goat cheese, divided
4 leeks, trimmed, cleaned, and thinly sliced
⅓ cup fresh basil, snipped

1. Heat 2 teaspoons of the oil in a cast-iron or steel skillet over high heat. Pat the tuna dry and sprinkle on each side with sea salt and black pepper.

2. When the oil is hot, carefully place the tuna in the pan. Sear the steaks on each side, turning once. Reduce the heat slightly and finish cooking the steaks, turning once. Transfer the fish to 4 plates. Spread each fillet with a portion of the goat cheese.

3. Heat the remaining 2 teaspoons of oil in the pan over high heat. When the oil is hot, add the leeks to the pan and sprinkle with sea salt. Cook until they are wilted, stirring constantly. Remove the pan from the heat and stir in the basil.

4. Divide the leeks among the 4 pieces of tuna and serve at once. Accompany with Garlic Mashed Potatoes (see page 273).

Cleaning Leeks

The tightly wrapped leaves of leeks hold dirt, which, if not cleaned, will ruin any meal. To clean leeks, begin by peeling away any discolored leaves and cutting off the top end, where it turns darker green. Then, starting about an inch from the base, slice the leeks in half lengthwise. Fill a bowl with cold water, fan the leeks slightly, and swish them around in the water, loosening any dirt with your fingers. Remove the leeks from the water and prepare them accordingly.

Roasted Cod with a White Bean and Dried-Tomato Ragu

Preparation: 20 minutes
Cooking: 10 minutes
Yield: 4 main-course servings

Mild-flavored cod is the perfect canvas for a hearty bean and tomato ragu. Quickly cooked leeks add an intriguing flavor to the dish. The ragu is enhanced with silken tofu to give the sauce a creamy texture and make the dish rich in phytoestrogens. Tips: Hake, monkfish, or striped bass can be substituted for the cod. The ragu can be prepared a day in advance without the tofu. The following day heat the ragu over low heat, adding more stock if necessary, to create a sauce. Stir in the pureed tofu just before serving.

1 cup dried tomatoes
1 cup boiling water
2 tablespoons olive oil, divided
4 cloves garlic, peeled and thinly sliced
1 cup dry white wine
1 15-ounce can white beans, drained and rinsed
2 cups homemade or canned low-sodium chicken broth
1½ pounds cod fillet
Sea salt to taste
Black pepper to taste
½ pound spinach, trimmed, washed, and drained
6 ounces silken tofu, pureed
2 leeks, trimmed, washed, and thinly sliced

1. Heat the oven to 425°F. Place the tomatoes in a bowl and pour the water on them. Allow them to macerate for 10 minutes. Drain the tomatoes. Thinly slice and set aside.

2. Heat 1 tablespoon of the olive oil in a Dutch oven over low heat. Add the garlic to the oil and cook until soft and fragrant, stirring occasionally.

3. Raise the heat to high and add the wine to the pot. Simmer for 2 minutes. Add the beans and dried tomatoes. Pour in

the chicken broth and bring to a boil. Reduce the heat and simmer for 10 minutes, stirring occasionally.

4. While the ragu is simmering, sprinkle the cod with sea salt and black pepper. Lightly oil a heavy baking tray. Place the fish on the tray and roast it for 10 minutes or until it is cooked through.

5. Remove the fish from the oven. Add the spinach to the ragu. Stir the ragu until the spinach wilts, approximately 1 minute.

6. Stir the silken tofu into the ragu and season with sea salt and black pepper.

7. Divide the ragu among 4 plates and place a portion of fish on each plate.

8. Heat the remaining olive oil in the Dutch oven over high heat. When the oil is hot, add the leeks to the pot. Sprinkle them with sea salt. Cook the leeks until they are soft and golden, stirring often, approximately 2 minutes. Garnish each portion of fish with the leeks and serve at once.

Chapter 18

Side Dishes and Accompaniments

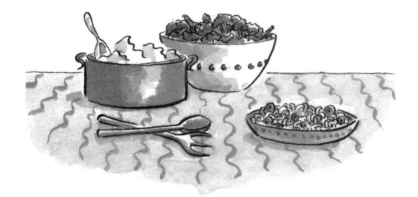

The versatility of soy is evident when it is paired with vegetables. Tofu, soy milk, and soy nuts can be used with a
variety of vegetables to create low-fat accompaniments that are
rich in antioxidants, phytoestrogens, and calcium. Soy can be
substituted for high-fat ingredients, such as cream, butter, and
mayonnaise, or combined with nonfat yogurt to make traditional fat-laden dishes significantly more healthful.

We have all gone to restaurants and ordered garlic mashed
potatoes and fussed about their heady flavor and creamy consistency. At the same time we knew the reason why they
tasted so good: cream and butter! Our Garlic Mashed Potatoes, loaded with phytoestrogens from soy milk and silken

tofu, have the same great flavor and texture but are much more nutritious. The Italian answer to mashed potatoes, Polenta, is in the same category. We love to eat it but always are wondering about the ingredients. Traditionally, butter and milk or cream are added at the end of cooking to enhance the flavor and consistency of the cornmeal. We add neither. We enrich it with tofu and soy milk to make a perfect menopause side dish. We suggest adding a small amount of creamy blue cheese as garnish. A little cheese is fine in a well-balanced diet.

Calcium-rich dishes also are represented here with what are becoming very popular cooking ingredients—dark leafy greens. Swiss Chard with Crisp Garlic and Pine Nuts is a delightful accompaniment. Earthy-tasting chard combines with sweet garlic and nutty pine nuts to create a dish rich in taste and nutrition. The Chinese cabbage bok choy, because of its pale color, is not often thought of as a calcium-rich vegetable, but with more than 100 milligrams in a 4-ounce cooked portion, it is a rich source. Although it is sometimes consumed raw, cooking it enhances its flavor and texture. Our quickly prepared Sesame Bok Choy is a wonderful way to enjoy this nutritious vegetable.

Cold vegetable salads also appear in this section. Elbow Macaroni Salad is a favorite picnic dish, but it is usually loaded with mayonnaise and offers little nutritionally except complex carbohydrates. We combine nonfat plain yogurt and tofu to create a phytoestrogen- and calcium-rich dressing. Green and black olives and cilantro provide the flavor.

Several dishes contain no soy and were created with the thought of using them as accompaniments to soy-based main courses. They are low in fat and high in flavor. Basmati Rice with Almonds and Raisins pairs beautifully with Curried Chickpeas, Tofu, and Arugula.

Hot or cold, the winning combination of soy and vegetables can't be beat.

Polenta

Preparation: 5 minutes
Cooking: 45 minutes
Yield: 4 side-dish servings

Made with coarsely ground cornmeal, polenta most often is served as an accompaniment to meat or vegetables. This version is made creamy by the addition of soy milk and silken tofu at the end of the cooking time. It is then dotted with blue cheese for a heavenly taste. Tips: No short cuts or quick methods are available for making polenta. It needs to be cooked for a full 45 minutes over low heat and stirred often. Shorter cooking time and less attention simply produces raw-tasting polenta. Leftover polenta is wonderful cut into squares, brushed with olive oil, and grilled or broiled.

4 cups water
Sea salt to taste
1 cup stone-ground yellow cornmeal
1 cup soy milk
4 ounces silken tofu, rinsed and pureed
Black pepper to taste
4 ounces Blue Castello cheese

1. Bring the water to a boil in a heavy-bottomed pan. Add sea salt. Slowly whisk in the cornmeal. When all the cornmeal has been added, stir the polenta with a wooden spoon for 2 more minutes.

2. Reduce the heat to low. Cook the polenta until it is creamy and no longer raw tasting, stirring every 5 minutes. The process will take approximately 45 minutes.

3. Stir in the soy milk and tofu. Season with sea salt and black pepper.

4. Divide the polenta among 4 plates and dot each serving with the cheese.

Garlic Mashed Potatoes

Garlic mashed potatoes are a restaurant side-dish staple. Generally made with cream and butter, they are a nutritional nightmare. Our version, which uses soy milk and silken tofu, is surprisingly rich and creamy, and it is a phytoestrogenic powerhouse. Tips: We always mash potatoes with a handheld masher. If you mash the potatoes with an electric mixer, don't overmix them, or they will be gooey. A few lumps are fine. Also, if you need to keep the potatoes warm, do so in a double boiler.

Preparation: 15 minutes
Cooking: 35 minutes
Yield: 6 side-dish servings

1½ cups soy milk
10 cloves garlic, peeled
6 ounces silken tofu, chopped
2½ pounds Yellow Finn potatoes, scrubbed
Sea salt to taste
Black pepper to taste
4 tablespoons flat-leaf parsley, chopped

1. Combine the soy milk and garlic in a saucepan. Gently bring the milk to a simmer. After 15 minutes add the tofu to the saucepan. Simmer the garlic cloves until tender, approximately another 10 minutes. Puree the mixture in a food processor or blender.

2. While the garlic cloves are simmering, place the potatoes in a Dutch oven and cover them with cold water. Bring the water to a boil, reduce the heat, and simmer the potatoes until tender, approximately 25 minutes.

3. Drain the potatoes and return them to the pot. Shake the potatoes over low heat to remove any excess moisture. Remove the pot from the heat.

4. Add the garlic-soy mixture to the potatoes. Mash the potatoes with a masher until they are smooth. Season with sea salt and black pepper. Transfer the potatoes to a large bowl, garnish with the parsley, and serve at once.

Spicy Soy Nuts

Preparation: 5 minutes

Cooking: 10 minutes

Yield: 1½ cups

Soy nuts are not typically thought of as a snack food, but they are delicious when cooked this way. Try these spicy soy nuts as a phyto-estrogen-rich snack, part of a quick breakfast or lunch on the go, or sprinkled on salads or cooked vegetables. Tip: *For the best flavor keep the nuts in a tightly sealed container.*

1½ cups soy nuts
1 teaspoon canola oil
½ teaspoon cayenne
¼ teaspoon sea salt

1. Heat the oven to 325°F. In a bowl combine the nuts, oil, cayenne, and salt. Transfer to a heavy baking sheet. Roast until they are fragrant, approximately 10 minutes.

2. Allow to cool. Store in a tightly sealed container.

Rosemary Roasted Potatoes

Preparation: 10 minutes

Cooking: 45 minutes

Yield: 6 side-dish servings

Fresh rosemary is fragrant and delicious when roasted with potatoes. In this low-fat dish, a light coating of olive oil and a hot oven produces potatoes with a crisp exterior and a soft and creamy interior. Tips: *Use a heavy-duty baking tray in this recipe. A lighter-weight tray, such as a cookie sheet, will cause the potatoes to burn. Also, an upside-down spatula is the best tool for scraping the potatoes off the tray.*

2½ pounds Yukon Gold or Yellow Finn potatoes, scrubbed
**   and cut into medium-sized cubes**
2 tablespoons extra-virgin olive oil
Sea salt to taste
Black pepper to taste
3 tablespoons fresh rosemary, chopped

1. Heat the oven to 400°F. Place the potatoes in a large bowl. Drizzle with olive oil and sprinkle with sea salt and black pepper.

2. Transfer the potatoes to 1 large or 2 smaller heavy baking trays and spread in a single layer. Place the tray(s) in the oven and roast the potatoes for 30 minutes. Sprinkle with rosemary and roast 15 minutes more.

3. Remove the potatoes from the oven and serve immediately.

Fresh Parsley and Romano Breadcrumbs

These breadcrumbs are wonderful on chicken, fish, vegetables, and even as a topping for pasta. Tip: *Save your leftover bread and make a double batch. They freeze well.*

Preparation: 10 minutes
Cooking: 0
Yield: 4 cups

4 cups tightly packed rustic bread cubes
4 tablespoons fresh flat-leaf parsley
4 tablespoons grated Romano cheese
1 tablespoon extra-virgin olive oil
Sea salt to taste
Black pepper to taste

1. Place the bread cubes, parsley, and Romano cheese in the work bowl of a food processor fitted with a metal blade.

2. Turn on the machine and drizzle in the olive oil. Process the ingredients until fine. Season with sea salt and black pepper. Use immediately or wrap tightly and freeze.

Braised Collard Greens with Raisins and Pine Nuts

Preparation: 10 minutes
Cooking: 20 minutes
Yield: 4 side-dish servings

Greens, which are a great source of antioxidants, are gaining popularity in the United States. This version is a medley of contrasts—earthy collard greens, sweet raisins, and crunchy pine nuts. Serve it with your favorite chicken or fish entrée. Tips: *This recipe works well with both kale and broccoli rabe. Broccoli rabe cooks in about half the time it takes to cook collards. Also, pine nuts have a tendency to burn quickly, so monitor them closely after 6 minutes.*

1 cup raisins
1 cup boiling water
¼ cup pine nuts
Sea salt to taste
1 tablespoon extra-virgin olive oil
2 cloves garlic, peeled and sliced
1 pound collard greens, trimmed, chopped, washed, and drained
Raisin-soaking water
Black pepper to taste

1. Place the raisins in a bowl. Pour the water over them and allow them to plump for 10 minutes. Drain the raisins and reserve their soaking water. Set the raisins and their soaking water aside.

2. Meanwhile, place the pine nuts in a small skillet and lightly sprinkle with sea salt. Toast them over very low heat, tossing often, until golden, approximately 6 minutes.

3. While the raisins are soaking and the pine nuts are toasting, heat the olive oil in a Dutch oven over low heat. Add the garlic to the pot and cook it until soft and fragrant, stirring often. Raise the heat to medium, add the collards to the pot,

and sprinkle with sea salt. Cover the pot, steam for 3 minutes, and then add the raisin-soaking water.

4. Bring the liquid to a boil, reduce the heat, and braise the collards until tender, approximately 15 minutes longer. Season with sea salt and black pepper.

5. Garnish the collards with the raisins and pine nuts. Divide them among four plates and serve immediately.

Basmati Rice with Almonds and Raisins

Sweet basmati rice pairs well with almonds and raisins. Try this side dish with Curried Chickpeas, Tofu, and Arugula for a heart-healthy and fiber-rich meal.

Preparation: 10 minutes
Cooking: 25 minutes
Yield: 4 side-dish servings

⅓ **cup slivered almonds**
Sea salt to taste
3 cups water
1½ cups basmati rice
1 cup raisins

1. Place the almonds in a small skillet and sprinkle with sea salt. Toast the almonds over low heat, tossing occasionally, until they are golden and fragrant.

2. While the almonds are toasting, bring the water to a boil in a saucepan. Stir the rice into the water. Return the water to a boil and cover the pan, leaving the lid slightly ajar.

3. Cook the rice for 15 minutes. Scatter the raisins on the rice. Cover the pan and cook the rice for 10 more minutes. Remove the pan from the heat and allow the rice to rest for 5 minutes.

4. Stir the rice with a fork and garnish with the almonds. Serve hot or at room temperature.

Israeli Couscous with Broccoli Rabe and Raisins

Preparation: 10
minutes
Cooking: 15 minutes
Yield: 4 side-dish
servings

Traditional North African couscous is a fine-grained food that is made with ground semolina and flour. The ingredients are blended and rolled until tiny pellets are formed. The Israeli variety is toasted and is larger than the traditional kind, making it heartier and a better absorber of flavors. This version is cooked with plump raisins and antioxidant-rich broccoli rabe, a delicious blend of contrasting flavors.

3 cups water
Sea salt to taste
1½ cups Israeli couscous
1 cup raisins
1 teaspoon olive oil
1 clove garlic, peeled and sliced
**12 ounces broccoli rabe, washed, drained, and finely
   chopped**
1 cup low-sodium canned chicken broth
1 tablespoon unsalted butter
Black pepper to taste

1. Bring the water to a boil in a medium-sized pot and add sea salt. Stir in the couscous and raisins. Reduce the heat and simmer until all of the liquid has evaporated and the couscous is tender, approximately 12 minutes.

2. While the couscous is cooking, heat the olive oil in a skillet over low heat. Add the garlic to the oil and cook until soft and fragrant. Raise the heat to high and add the broccoli rabe. Sprinkle the rabe with sea salt and cook for 2 minutes.

3. Add the chicken broth to the skillet and bring to a boil. Add the butter and cover the skillet. Cook the rabe for 5 more minutes.

4. When the couscous is tender, stir the broccoli rabe into the pot. Season with sea salt and black pepper.

5. Transfer the couscous to a bowl and serve at once.

Broccoli with Oyster Sauce and Soy Nuts

Broccoli with oyster sauce is a common Asian dish. We have garnished it with Spicy Soy Nuts, which increases the phytoestrogen content and adds a pleasant crunch to the dish. Broccoli is an excellent source of nondairy calcium. Tip: *To prepare the broccoli for this recipe, trim 1 inch off the bottom of each stem. Separate the stems from the flowers. Cut the flowers into 1-inch pieces. Peel the stems and slice them into disks.*

Preparation: 15 minutes
Cooking: 15 minutes
Yield: 4 side-dish servings

1½ cups water
Sea salt to taste
1½ pounds broccoli, trimmed, stems and florets separated, stems peeled and sliced into disks
2 tablespoons shoyu or tamari
1 tablespoon dark miso
2 tablespoons oyster sauce
¼ cup low-sodium chicken broth or water
1 teaspoon sugar
1 teaspoon sesame oil
Broccoli-steaming water
1 tablespoon canola oil
1 1-inch piece gingerroot, peeled and minced
3 cloves garlic, peeled and sliced
⅓ cup Spicy Soy Nuts (see page 274)

1. Bring the water to a boil in a Dutch oven and add sea salt. Add the broccoli disks to the water and cover the pot. Steam for 2 minutes. Add the florets and cover the pot. Steam the broccoli for 4 minutes or until tender. Drain the broccoli, reserving the steaming water. Set the water aside. Cool the broccoli under running water and set it aside.

2. While the broccoli is steaming, prepare the sauce by whisking together in a medium-sized bowl the shoyu, miso,

oyster sauce, chicken broth or water, sugar, sesame oil, and broccoli-steaming water.

3. Heat the oil in a wok over high heat. When the oil is hot, add the gingerroot and garlic to the wok and cook for 30 seconds.

4. Add the broccoli to the wok and toss it. Cook the broccoli for 1 minute. Whisk the sauce and add it to the wok. Cook the broccoli until hot.

5. Transfer the broccoli to a large platter and garnish with Spicy Soy Nuts.

Monique's New Potatoes with Cucumber Raita

Preparation: 10 minutes
Cooking: 25 minutes
Yield: 3 cups

A raita is an Indian-inspired yogurt-mint sauce. Yogurt, potatoes, and mint complement each other, and the cucumber adds just the right crunch and coolness to the dish. Our neighbor, Monique Spencer, gave us this recipe, and we added silken tofu to increase the phytoestrogen content. Tips: *This recipe makes more than enough raita to serve with the potatoes. Use the extra as a salad dressing or in place of mayonnaise on your favorite sandwich. Also, since the raita's flavor improves with an overnight chill, consider making it a day in advance.*

24 ounces nonfat plain yogurt
6 ounces silken tofu, pureed
1 cucumber, peeled, seeded, and diced
2 plum tomatoes, diced
1 small clove garlic, peeled and minced
2 scallions, trimmed and thinly sliced
3 tablespoons sesame tahini
¼ cup fresh mint, chopped
Sea salt to taste
Black pepper to taste
2 pounds small new potatoes, scrubbed

1. Combine the yogurt, tofu, cucumber, tomatoes, garlic, scallions, tahini, and mint in a nonmetal bowl. Season with sea salt and black pepper. Cover the raita and refrigerate while the potatoes cook.

2. Place the potatoes in a Dutch oven and cover with cold water. Bring the water to a boil. Reduce the heat and simmer the potatoes until tender, approximately 20 minutes.

3. Drain the potatoes and return them to the Dutch oven. Shake the potatoes over low heat to rid them of all their moisture.

4. Transfer the potatoes to a serving bowl. Stir 2 cups of the raita into the potatoes and serve immediately.

Swiss Chard with Crisp Garlic and Pine Nuts

Many of Hope's patients want to cook more with greens for their nutritional and antioxidant properties but are not sure how to do it. This is a straightforward preparation that can be adapted to other greens, such as red chard, spinach, broccoli rabe, dandelion greens, or arugula.

This dish was inspired by a popular recipe—Pasta with Swiss Chard and Pine Nuts in our previous cookbook, The Pregnancy Cookbook. *Swiss chard and pine nuts go together well, complementing and bringing out their respective flavors. The fried garlic is sweet and delicious.* Tip: *The garlic can be cooked and the pine nuts toasted earlier in the day and left at room temperature.*

Preparation: 15 minutes
Cooking: 15 minutes
Yield: 4 side-dish servings

4 tablespoons pine nuts
Sea salt to taste
1 tablespoon extra-virgin olive oil
8 large cloves garlic, peeled and quartered
1 pound Swiss chard, washed, drained, and trimmed, stems sliced into matchsticks and leaves coarsely chopped
1 cup water
Black pepper to taste

1. Place the pine nuts in a small skillet over low heat and sprinkle with sea salt. Toast until golden, approximately 7 minutes. Toss often to prevent them from burning. Transfer to a plate.

2. While the pine nuts are toasting, heat the olive oil in a wok over low heat. Add the garlic to the oil and sprinkle with sea salt. Cook the garlic until golden and very soft, turning occasionally, approximately 15 minutes. Remove the garlic from the wok and set aside.

3. Raise the heat to high under the wok. Add the chard to the wok and cook for 3 minutes, stirring often. Add the water. Cover the wok and braise the chard until it is tender, stirring occasionally. Season with sea salt and black pepper.

4. Transfer the chard to a large platter and garnish with the pine nuts and garlic.

Sesame Bok Choy

Preparation: 5 minutes
Cooking: 10 minutes
Yield: 4 side-dish servings

Bok choy is a Chinese green making its way into mainstream cooking. Like Swiss chard, it is prized for its sweet and crisp stems and earthy-tasting leaves; and like many greens, it is a nutritional powerhouse, packed with calcium and fiber. Tip: *This preparation also works well with spinach and broccoli. If you use broccoli, steam it first in 1 cup of water; reserve the steaming water for use in the sauce.*

1 tablespoon sesame oil
1 1-inch piece gingerroot, peeled and minced
2 cloves garlic, peeled and sliced
1 pound bok choy, trimmed, stems sliced diagonally into
**   ¾-inch-thick pieces and leaves coarsely chopped**
1 cup vegetable broth or water
Sea salt to taste
Black pepper to taste
4 tablespoons toasted sesame seeds

1. Heat the oil in a wok over low heat. Add the gingerroot and garlic and cook until soft and fragrant.

2. Raise the heat to high. When the wok is hot, add the bok choy to it. Cook the bok choy for 1 minute, stirring constantly.

3. Add the vegetable broth or water to the wok and bring the liquid to a boil. Reduce the heat and simmer the bok choy until tender, approximately 6 minutes.

4. Season the bok choy with sea salt and black pepper. Transfer to a serving platter and garnish with sesame seeds. It can be served hot or at room temperature.

Spicy Brown Rice

Brown rice is an excellent source of fiber. This dish can accompany your favorite entrée or be used as a filling for a burrito or roll-up sandwich. Add 12 ounces of cubed, firm tofu in step 2 to turn the dish into a main course. Tip: *If you can't locate brown basmati rice, use a medium-grain brown rice.*

Preparation: 10 minutes
Cooking: 40 minutes
Yield: 4 side-dish servings

1 tablespoon canola oil
3 cloves garlic, peeled and sliced
1 onion, peeled and diced
1 green bell pepper, cored and diced
1½ teaspoons chili powder
1 teaspoon ground cumin
½ teaspoon coriander
½ teaspoon oregano
½ teaspoon cayenne
3½ cups water
1 tomato, diced
Sea salt to taste
Black pepper to taste
1½ cups brown basmati rice

1. Heat the canola oil in a Dutch oven over low heat. Add the garlic and cook until soft. Add the onion and cook until soft. Add the bell pepper and cook until it begins to soften.

2. Add the chili powder, cumin, coriander, oregano, and cayenne and cook for 2 minutes. Raise the heat to high and add the water. Add the tomato and bring the broth to a boil. Season with sea salt and black pepper.

3. Stir the rice into the pot and return the broth to a boil. Reduce the heat and cover the pot, leaving the lid slightly ajar. Simmer until all of the liquid is absorbed and the rice is tender, approximately 30 minutes.

4. Fluff the rice with a fork. It can be served immediately or at room temperature.

Elbow Macaroni Salad

Preparation: 15 minutes
Cooking: 10 minutes
Chilling: 2 hours
Yield: 4 side-dish servings

Traditional macaroni salad contains a great deal of mayonnaise. This version features nonfat yogurt and silken tofu in place of the mayonnaise, making it low in fat and high in calcium and phytoestrogens—a perfect menopause recipe. Tip: *The salad can be prepared a day in advance. Not only is this convenient, but also the overnight chill will give the flavors time to fully develop.*

DRESSING

1½ cups plain nonfat yogurt
1 tablespoon sugar
1 small clove garlic, peeled and minced
2 tablespoons tahini
1 teaspoon Dijon mustard
6 ounces silken tofu
Sea salt to taste
Black pepper to taste

SALAD

Sea salt to taste
12 ounces elbow macaroni
4 eggs
6 Sicilian olives, pitted and chopped
12 Kalamata olives, pitted and chopped
1 cucumber, peeled, seeded, and diced
3 plum tomatoes, diced
½ cup cilantro, chopped
Black pepper to taste

1. Bring a large pot of water to a boil. Add sea salt to the water, followed by the macaroni and eggs. Cook the pasta until tender. Drain the macaroni and cool under running water. Set aside. Separate and chop the egg whites.

2. While the pasta is cooking, combine the yogurt, sugar, garlic, tahini, mustard, and tofu in the work bowl of a food processor fitted with a metal blade. Process until a creamy dressing is formed. Season with sea salt and black pepper. Set aside.

3. Place the macaroni in a large serving bowl. Add the 2 varieties of olives, cucumber, tomatoes, egg whites, and cilantro to the bowl. Add the dressing to the salad. Stir the salad thoroughly and season with sea salt and black pepper. Cover the bowl and refrigerate for at least 2 hours.

Chapter 19

Sweets and Goodies

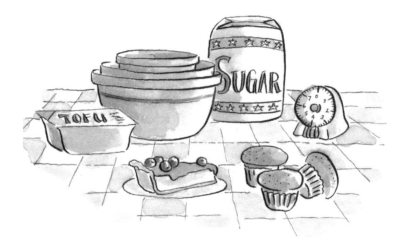

T hanks to the wonderful versatility of phytoestrogen-rich
flaxseed and soy, desserts now can fit perfectly into a
healthful diet. Soy and flaxseed desserts are low in fat and rich
in phytoestrogens, calcium, fiber, and protein.

It is just as easy baking with flaxseed and soy as cooking
with it. You will need to make only one change in your
baking. Because of the high moisture content of flaxseed
and soy, your baked goods now will need to bake at a lower
temperature. Too high a temperature will result in under-
done food. Flaxseed-laced baking produces moist brownies
and cookies and crunchy toppings. Silken tofu makes deca-

dent puddings, cheesecakes, and sauces. Soy milk replaces cow's milk in yeast and quick breads to produce a tender crust.

You have no reason to skip dessert now when you can indulge in our rich Chocolate-Orange Cheesecake. With flaxseed in the crust and silken tofu in the filling, it is overflowing with phytoestrogens yet relatively low in fat. When that chocolate craving overwhelms you, reach for our delectable brownies. Their moistness comes from flaxseed and soy milk, and they contain no eggs or butter. Do you need a little pick-me-up before going to the gym? Pass on those ubiquitous energy bars and try our Estro Bars instead. They are packed with dried fruit, fruit juice, flaxseed, and oats. They are designed to provide you with sustained energy and phytoestrogens on the run.

So the next time your sweet tooth begins aching, don't deny yourself because you are following a phytoestrogen-rich diet. Alleviate the pain with one of our goodies.

Malted Vanilla Pudding

Malted vanilla ice cream is a real treat. Here are the same flavors in a soy-based pudding.

Preparation: 5 minutes
Cooking: 0
Yield: 4 servings

12 ounces silken tofu
1½ teaspoons vanilla
3 tablespoons malt syrup
6 tablespoons maple syrup

1. Place the tofu, vanilla, malt syrup, and maple syrup in the work bowl of a food processor fitted with a metal blade. Blend until a smooth pudding forms.

2. Divide the pudding among 4 dessert cups. Serve immediately or cover the cups and refrigerate.

Chocolate Pudding

*Preparation: 5
minutes
Cooking: 0
Yield: 4 servings*

Silken tofu makes creamy desserts without the fat and calories of cream-based dairy products. You get an unbeatable combination of great taste and great nutrition. Tip: *If you like your pudding sweeter, stir in more maple syrup after the pudding has been blended.*

12 ounces silken tofu
2½ tablespoons unsweetened cocoa powder
6 tablespoons maple syrup
3 tablespoons brown-rice syrup
1 teaspoon vanilla extract

1. Place the tofu, cocoa powder, maple syrup, brown-rice syrup, and vanilla in the work bowl of a food processor fitted with a metal blade. Blend until a smooth pudding forms.
2. Divide the pudding among 4 dessert cups. Serve immediately or cover the cups and refrigerate.

Dried Cherry–Chocolate Muffins

*Preparation: 15
minutes
Cooking: 18 minutes
Yield: 12 muffins*

Beware of store-bought muffins—they can be as high in fat and calories as cake. This low-fat version uses no added fat and contains a healthful dose of phytoestrogens from the soy milk and flaxseed. Tips: *In a muffin recipe, when combining the wet and dry ingredients, it is important to fold them together gently. If the batter is vigorously mixed, the muffins will be tough. Also, if dried cherries are not available, other dried fruits, such as blueberries, strawberries, or cranberries, are fine substitutes.*

⅓ cup flaxseed

Canola oil for greasing the muffin tray

1 cup dried (pitted) cherries

1 cup soy milk

1¾ cups unbleached, all-purpose flour

¾ cup raw sugar plus additional sugar for sprinkling on top

2 teaspoons baking powder

1 teaspoon baking soda

¼ teaspoon salt

2 eggs

8 ounces chocolate chips

1. Heat the oven to 350°F. Place the flaxseed in an electric coffee grinder and grind until it resembles flour.

2. Lightly grease 12 muffin cups with canola oil. Place the cherries in a bowl and pour the soy milk on them. Set aside.

3. In a large mixing bowl, stir together the flour, ¾ cup of the sugar, baking powder, baking soda, salt, and ground flaxseed. Set the bowl aside.

4. Whisk the eggs into the soy milk-cherry mixture.

5. Pour liquid ingredients into dry ingredients and add chocolate chips to the batter. Gently fold ingredients together.

6. Fill each muffin tin approximately 2/3 full with batter. Sprinkle sugar on each muffin. Bake the muffins for 18 minutes or until they are golden. Allow the muffins to cool before removing them from the tin.

Blueberry-Banana Muffins

Everyone has a favorite blueberry muffin recipe. Our version contains a banana for sweetness and tofu. Tofu is not an ingredient usually found in quick bread recipes, but besides the phytoestrogens it adds, it also produces a moist muffin.

Preparation: 15 minutes
Cooking: 18 minutes
Yield: 12 muffins

1 cup soy milk

1 egg

4 ounces silken tofu

1 ripe banana

1 tablespoon canola oil plus additional oil for oiling the muffin tray

2 cups unbleached, all-purpose flour

1 cup raw sugar plus additional sugar for sprinkling on the muffins

2 teaspoons baking powder

1 teaspoon baking soda

¼ teaspoon salt

1 cup fresh or frozen blueberries

1. Heat the oven to 350°F. Combine the milk, egg, tofu, banana, and oil in the work bowl of a food processor fitted with a metal blade. Process the ingredients until smooth. Set the work bowl aside.

2. In a large mixing bowl, stir together the flour, 1 cup of sugar, baking powder, baking soda, and salt.

3. Pour the liquid ingredients into the dry. Add the blueberries to the batter. Gently fold the ingredients together.

4. Lightly oil 12 muffin tins with canola oil. Fill each muffin tin approximately 2/3 full with batter. Sprinkle sugar on each muffin. Bake the muffins for 18 minutes or until they are golden. Allow the muffins to cool before removing them from the tin.

Soda Bread

Preparation: 10 minutes
Cooking: 40 minutes
Yield: 1 loaf

This menopause adaptation of a traditional Irish soda bread contains flaxseed, soy milk, and yogurt, so it is rich in phytoestrogens and calcium. A portion of the flour is whole wheat in order to increase the fiber content. Try it for breakfast or a snack. Tip: *As with all quick breads, be certain not to overmix the ingredients. Stir the wet and dry ingredients together only until they are blended.*

½ cup flax plus 2 tablespoons flaxseed
2 teaspoons canola oil
2 cups unbleached, white flour
½ cup whole-wheat flour
½ cup raw sugar
2 teaspoons baking powder
1 teaspoon baking soda
1 teaspoon sea salt
2 cups currants
2 eggs
1¾ cups plain nonfat yogurt

1. Grind ½ cup of the flaxseed in a coffee grinder until it resembles flour. Set it aside. Oil the bottom and sides of a 10-inch cast-iron skillet. Heat the oven to 350°F.

2. In a large bowl stir together the unbleached flour, whole-wheat flour, ground and whole flaxseed, sugar, baking powder, baking soda, sea salt, and currants.

3. In another bowl whisk together the eggs and yogurt. Add to the dry ingredients and mix the ingredients until they are combined.

4. Transfer the batter to the prepared skillet. Cut an X into the batter.

5. Place the skillet in the oven and bake the bread until it is done, approximately 40 minutes.

6. Allow the bread to cool for 15 minutes in the skillet and transfer to a wire rack to finish cooling. Slice the bread and spread it with an all-fruit jam.

Chocolate–Peanut Butter Cookies

Preparation: 10 minutes
Cooking: 18 minutes
Yield: 20 cookies

Adding peanut butter to a chocolate chip cookie recipe gives the cookies a chewy texture. Flaxseed and soy milk provide the phytoestrogens in this sweet menopause treat that everyone will enjoy. Tips: *When forming the cookies, flour your hands lightly. It will make the job much easier. Also, the dough freezes well and can be baked later.*

2 cups unbleached, all-purpose flour

1 cup raw sugar

2 teaspoons baking powder

1 teaspoon baking soda

½ teaspoon salt

⅔ cup flaxseed

1 cup freshly ground peanut butter

⅓ cup blackstrap molasses

2 eggs

1 teaspoon vanilla extract

1 cup soy milk

8 ounces semisweet chocolate chips

1. Heat the oven to 300°F. In a large bowl whisk together the flour, sugar, baking powder, baking soda, and salt. Set the bowl aside.

2. Grind the flaxseed in a coffee mill until it resembles flour. In another bowl combine the peanut butter, molasses, and ground flaxseed. Set the bowl aside.

3. In another bowl whisk together the eggs, vanilla, and soy milk. Whisk this mixture into the peanut butter mixture.

4. Add the dry ingredients to the wet. Stir in the chocolate chips.

5. Lightly flour your hands. Form the dough into approximately 20 2-inch balls. Place the balls on a heavy sheet pan. Bake the cookies for 18 minutes or until they are done.

6. Allow the cookies to cool. Transfer them to an airtight container.

Cranberry–Orange Cloud Cookies

These cookies are the result of a scone recipe that went awry. The final product still looked and tasted fine, so we decided to include the recipe. Not dense like cookies or airy like scones, these cookies fall somewhere in between. They are a good source of calcium and phytoestrogens. Tip: *As with making muffins and scones, when preparing these cookies, use full, even strokes when combining the wet and dry ingredients. Take care not to overmix the batter.*

Preparation: 10 minutes
Cooking: 18 minutes
Yield: 20 cookies

½ **cup flaxseed**
2 cups unbleached, all-purpose flour
1 cup raw sugar plus additional sugar for sprinkling
2 teaspoons baking powder
1 teaspoon baking soda
½ **teaspoon salt**
1½ **cups plain nonfat yogurt**
2 eggs, divided
1 tablespoon orange juice concentrate, thawed
1 cup dried cranberries

1. Heat the oven to 325°F. Grind the flaxseed in a coffee grinder until it resembles flour. In a large bowl stir together the flour, sugar, baking powder, baking soda, salt, and ground flaxseed. Set the bowl aside.

2. In another bowl, whisk together the yogurt, 1 egg, and the orange juice concentrate.

3. Make a well in the dry ingredients and stir the wet ingredients into it, along with the cranberries.

4. With a large spoon, drop approximately 2-inch portions of the batter onto a heavy baking tray. Beat the remaining egg. Brush each cookie with the egg and sprinkle with sugar. Bake the cookies for 18 minutes or until they are done. Allow them to cool before transferring to an airtight container.

Apple and Rhubarb Crisp

Preparation: 20 minutes
Cooking: 1 hour
Yield: 6 servings

While searching for calcium-rich ingredients, we were pleasantly surprised to find rhubarb included. When combined with apples, it makes a delectable dessert. In addition, our crisp topping contains flaxseed and soy nuts, making this treat a phytoestrogen powerhouse. Tip: When selecting rhubarb, choose firm stalks with no brownish edges. Thin stalks are more tender and less bitter. If only thick stalks are available, peel them.

FILLING

- 1 pound rhubarb, trimmed and cut into 1-inch pieces, ½-inch wide
- 2 pounds Cortland or other cooking apples, cored and cut into 2-inch pieces
- 1 cup raw sugar
- 1½ teaspoons ground cinnamon
- 3 tablespoons unbleached, all-purpose flour

TOPPING

- ⅓ cup flaxseed
- 1 cup rolled oats
- ⅓ cup brown sugar
- ½ teaspoon ground cinnamon
- ⅓ cup soy nuts, ground
- ¼ cup honey, warmed

1. Heat the oven to 325°F. To prepare the filling, combine the rhubarb and apples in a large bowl. Stir in the sugar, cinnamon, and flour. Transfer the filling to a 2-quart baking dish. Set aside.

2. Grind the flaxseed in a coffee grinder until it resembles flour. To prepare the topping, stir together the rolled oats, brown sugar, cinnamon, soy nuts, and ground flaxseed in a bowl. Drizzle in the honey and stir the ingredients until well combined.

3. Spread the topping on the filling. Bake the crisp until the fruit is bubbling and the topping is golden, approximately 1 hour.

4. Allow the crisp to cool slightly before serving. If desired, accompany the crisp with vanilla frozen yogurt.

Blueberry Crisp

This is one of our favorite desserts, especially when fresh blueberries are abundant and inexpensive. During other times of the year, we use frozen blueberries. The slightly sweet crisp topping contains plenty of phytoestrogens from the flaxseed and soy nuts. To increase the amount of phytoestrogens, accompany the crisp with Creamy Vanilla-Maple Sauce (see page 302).

Preparation: 20 minutes
Cooking: 1 hour
Yield: 6 servings

FILLING
6 cups fresh or frozen blueberries
Juice from 1 lemon
½ cup raw sugar
2 tablespoons unbleached, all-purpose flour

TOPPING
½ cup flaxseed
1 cup rolled oats
½ cup toasted wheat germ
⅓ cup brown sugar
⅓ cup soy nuts, ground
¼ cup honey
¼ cup brown-rice syrup
1 tablespoon vanilla extract

1. Heat the oven to 325°F. To prepare the filling, place the blueberries in a large bowl. Sprinkle them with the lemon juice, sugar, and flour. Gently toss the filling. Transfer to a 2-quart baking dish. Set it aside.

2. Grind the flaxseed in a coffee grinder until it resembles flour. To prepare the topping, stir together the rolled oats, wheat germ, brown sugar, soy nuts, and ground flaxseed in a bowl.

3. Combine the honey and brown-rice syrup in a small saucepan. Gently heat until warm. Stir in the vanilla extract.

4. Pour the honey mixture into the flaxseed mixture and stir the ingredients until well combined.

5. Spread the topping on the filling. Bake the crisp until the fruit is bubbling and the topping is golden, approximately 1 hour.

6. Allow the crisp to cool slightly before serving. If desired, accompany with Creamy Vanilla-Maple Sauce (see page 302).

Brownies

Preparation: 10 minutes
Cooking: 25 minutes
Yield: 16 brownies

With soy milk and flaxseed as the major ingredients of these phytoestrogen-rich brownies, it will be difficult to feel guilty about eating them. This recipe makes cakelike brownies, not chewy ones.

Canola oil for oiling baking pan
½ cup flaxseed
1½ cups unbleached, all-purpose flour
½ cup unsweetened cocoa powder
1 cup raw sugar
2 teaspoons baking soda
1 cup soy milk
1 teaspoon vanilla extract
4 tablespoons brown-rice syrup
4 ounces vanilla yogurt

1. Heat the oven to 325°F. Lightly oil an 8 x 8–inch baking pan.

2. Grind the flaxseed in a coffee grinder until it resembles flour. Set aside.

3. Combine the flour, cocoa, sugar, and baking soda in a large bowl.

4. Combine the soy milk, ground flaxseed, vanilla, brown-rice syrup, and yogurt in the work bowl of a food processor

fitted with a metal blade. Process the ingredients until they bubble.

5. Fold the liquid ingredients into the dry ingredients. Spoon the batter into the prepared pan. Bake the brownies for 25 minutes or until a toothpick inserted into the center comes out clean.

6. Remove the brownies from the oven and allow them to cool before slicing them.

Gingerbread

Fresh ginger adds a clean, intense flavor to this popular treat. The large amount of flaxseed not only provides phytoestrogens but also produces an incredibly moist gingerbread.

Preparation: 15 minutes
Cooking: 35 minutes
Yield: 18 pieces

Canola oil for baking pan
2 cups unbleached, all-purpose flour
1 teaspoon baking soda
1 teaspoon baking powder
2 teaspoons cinnamon
½ teaspoon salt
⅔ cup flaxseed
1 egg
1 cup dark molasses
1 cup soy milk
1 4-inch piece gingerroot, peeled and minced
1 cup raisins

1. Heat the oven to 325°F. Lightly oil a 9 x 9-inch baking pan and set aside.

2. In a large bowl whisk together the flour, baking soda, baking powder, cinnamon, and salt. Set the bowl aside.

3. Grind the flaxseed in a coffee grinder until it resembles flour. Place the egg, molasses, soy milk, gingerroot, and ground flaxseed into the work bowl of a food processor fitted with a

metal blade. Process the ingredients until well combined.

4. Pour the liquid ingredients into the dry ingredients and stir until they are combined. Stir the raisins into the batter.

5. Transfer the batter to the prepared pan. Bake the ginger-bread for 30 to 35 minutes or until a toothpick inserted into the center emerges clean. Allow the gingerbread to cool before cutting it.

Estro Bars

Preparation: 15 minutes
Cooking: 18 minutes
Yield: 9 bars

These delicious snack bars are akin to the carbohydrate-rich bars on the market for endurance athletes. Our version tastes similar yet is rich in phytoestrogens from the flaxseed and soy nuts in the bars. They are flavored with peanuts and peaches.

½ cup peach juice concentrate
½ cup brown-rice syrup
8 dates, pitted and chopped
8 dried figs, chopped
3 tablespoons soy nuts
2 tablespoons sesame seeds
2/3 cup flaxseed
2 tablespoons natural peanut butter
2 cups rolled oats
1 cup rice-crisp cereal
1 teaspoon baking powder

1. Heat the oven to 350°F. Combine the peach juice concentrate and brown-rice syrup in a small saucepan. Gently heat until warm. Set the liquid aside.

2. Place the dates, figs, soy nuts, and sesame seeds in the work bowl of a food processor fitted with a metal blade. Process until they resemble paste. Leave the ingredients in the work bowl.

3. Grind the flaxseed in a coffee grinder until it resembles flour. Add the flaxseed and peanut butter to the work bowl and process for 20 seconds. Transfer to a large mixing bowl.

4. Place the oats, crisp cereal, and baking powder in the work bowl. Process for 10 seconds. Transfer to the mixing bowl and combine all of the ingredients well.

5. Pour the peach-syrup mixture into the mixing bowl and stir the ingredients thoroughly. Spread the dough into a 9 x 9-inch baking pan. Bake for 18 minutes.

6. Remove the pan from the oven and allow to cool. Cut the Estro Bars into 9 pieces. When they are cool, wrap them individually and store in the refrigerator.

Estro Bars II

Dried figs, oat bran, and oatmeal make these apple-flavored bars fiber rich. The healthful amounts of flaxseed and soy nuts make them the ideal "on the go" menopause snack. Tip: *The most efficient method for combining the dried fruit–nut–seed–cereal mixture is with your fingertips.*

Preparation: 15 minutes
Cooking: 18 minutes
Yield: 9 bars

⅔ cup flaxseed
½ cup apple-raspberry juice concentrate
⅔ cup brown-rice syrup
2 tablespoons malt syrup
½ cup raisins
8 dried figs, chopped
2 cups dried apple rings
¼ cup soy nuts
¼ cup sunflower seeds
2 cups rolled oats
1 cup rice-crisp cereal
1 teaspoon baking powder
3 tablespoons oat bran

1. Heat the oven to 350°F. Grind the flaxseed in a coffee grinder until it resembles flour. Set aside.

2. Combine the apple-raspberry juice concentrate, brown-rice syrup, and malt syrup in a small saucepan. Gently heat until warm.

3. Place the raisins, figs, and apple rings in the work bowl of a food processor fitted with a metal blade. Process until the ingredients form a ball, approximately 1 minute. Transfer to a large mixing bowl.

4. Place the soy nuts and sunflower seeds in the work bowl and process until coarsely chopped. Transfer to the mixing bowl.

5. Place the oats, crisp cereal, and baking powder in the work bowl and process for 10 seconds. Transfer to the mixing bowl and add the ground flaxseed and oat bran. Combine the ingredients thoroughly.

6. Pour the juice-syrup mixture into the mixing bowl and stir the ingredients until they are well combined. Spread the dough into a 9 x 9-inch baking pan. Bake the dough for 18 minutes.

7. Remove the pan from the oven and allow it to cool. Cut the Estro Bars into 9 pieces. When they are cool, wrap them individually and store in the refrigerator.

Chocolate–Orange Cheesecake

Preparation: 10 minutes
Cooking: 50 minutes
Chilling: 8 hours
Yield: 2 9-inch cakes

Silken tofu is the best tofu for making cheesecakes. When you combine it with soy cream cheese, you can make a great-tasting and healthful cheesecake without dairy cream cheese and eggs. Tips: You will need to plan ahead; the cheesecake needs an overnight chill. Also, if your cheesecake cracks while it is in the oven, don't fret—cover it with fresh berries.

CRUST

⅓ cup flaxseed

1½ cups graham cracker crumbs

5 tablespoons orange marmalade

FILLING

1¾ pounds silken tofu

1 cup raw sugar

6 tablespoons maple syrup

12 ounces soy cream cheese

½ cup unsweetened cocoa powder

2 teaspoons vanilla extract

1 teaspoon orange extract

1. Heat the oven to 300°F. To make the crust, grind the flaxseed in a coffee grinder until it resembles flour. Transfer to a bowl and stir in the graham cracker crumbs. Add the marmalade and with a spoon blend to make a dough. Press the dough into a thin layer in two 9-inch pie plates. Bake the crusts for 7 minutes. Remove from the oven and allow to cool while you prepare the filling.

2. To make the filling, place the tofu in the work bowl of a food processor fitted with a metal blade and process until smooth.

3. Add the sugar, maple syrup, soy cream cheese, cocoa, vanilla, and orange extract to the work bowl. Process the ingredients until smooth. If necessary, scrape down the bowl.

4. Divide the filling among the 2 crusts. Bake the cheesecakes for 40 to 50 minutes. Turn off the oven and leave them in the oven for 30 minutes.

5. Remove cheesecakes from the oven and allow to cool at room temperature.

6. Chill the cheesecakes for 8 hours. If desired, top with fresh berries.

Strawberry–Orange Sauce

Preparation: 5 minutes
Cooking: 20 minutes
Yield: 2 cups

This versatile sauce is wonderful drizzled on frozen yogurt, mixed into granola, or as a topping for a plain cheesecake. The creaminess comes from silken tofu.

2 cups frozen strawberries
½ cup orange juice
½ teaspoon orange extract
6 tablespoons sugar
5 ounces silken tofu

1. Combine the strawberries and orange juice in a medium-sized saucepan. Bring to a simmer and cook for 10 minutes.

2. Add the orange extract and sugar to the pan and simmer the sauce for 10 more minutes or until thick.

3. Transfer the sauce to the work bowl of a food processor fitted with metal blade. Add the tofu to the work bowl and process until a smooth sauce forms. Transfer to a bowl and cover. Chill the sauce.

Creamy Vanilla–Maple Sauce

Preparation: 5 minutes
Cooking: 10 minutes
Yield: 1 cup

This phytoestrogen-rich sauce makes a wonderful topping for crisps, puddings, or hot chocolate. One taste of this, and you will forget all about whipped cream.

½ cup soy milk
8 vanilla beans
8 ounces silken tofu
1¼ tablespoons vanilla extract
4 tablespoons maple syrup
3 tablespoons brown-rice syrup

1. Combine the soy milk and vanilla beans in a small saucepan. Gently heat. When ingredients are warm, remove from the heat. Allow to rest for 10 minutes. Remove the beans from the milk and discard them.

2. Transfer the soy milk to a food processor fitted with a metal blade. Add the tofu, vanilla extract, maple syrup, and brown-rice syrup to the work bowl. Process the ingredients until they are smooth and creamy. If necessary, stop the machine and scrape the bits of tofu that cling to the side of the bowl back toward the blade.

3. Transfer the sauce to a bowl and refrigerate until needed.

Index

chicken (continued)
    broth, canned, 195
    with cilantro and scallions, **244–45**
    curried bok choy and, **248–49**
    lemon-ginger tofu and, **246–48**
    ragu, **245–46**
    with tempeh, white beans, tomatoes, and basil, **249–51**
    two-mustard, **242–43**
    whole-wheat penne with asparagus, lemon and, **197–98**
chickpea(s):
    curried tofu, arugula and, **227–28**
    and lentil soup with root vegetables and couscous, Kate's, **125–27**
    and tofu patties with a yogurt-chili sauce, **219–21**
chili:
    tempeh, zucchini, and beef, **135–37**
    -yogurt sauce, tofu and chickpea patties with, **219–21**
Chinese food, 85–86
chocolate:
    cinnamon granola, **118–19**
    -dried cherry muffins, **288–89**
    frappé, **104**
    -orange cheesecake, **300–301**
    -peanut butter cookies, **292**
    pudding, **287–88**
cholesterol, blood, 24, 41–43, 68, 75
    dietary cholesterol and, 41–42
    HRT and, 51, 69
    levels of, 41–42
    as risk factor for heart disease, 42–43
    soy foods for lowering of, 31–32
    trans fatty acids and, 40
    see also high-density lipoprotein (HDL) cholesterol; low-density lipoprotein (LDL) cholesterol
cilantro:
    and arugula pesto, **148–49**
    chicken with scallions and, **244–45**
    linguine with corn, tofu and, **205–6**
cinnamon chocolate granola, **118–19**
citrus delight, **103**

clams, littleneck, linguine with spicy sausage, tomatoes and, **181–82**
cocoa, hot, **107–8**
cod:
    baked, with tomatoes and breadcrumbs, **262–63**
    roasted, with a white bean and dried-tomato ragu, **268–69**
collard greens:
    braised, with raisins and pine nuts, **276–77**
    kale and potato soup, **127–28**
colon cancer, 30, 31, 73
complex carbohydrates, 36–38
conjugated equine estrogens (Premarin), 48
cookies:
    chocolate-peanut butter, **292**
    cranberry-orange cloud, **293**
corn:
    farfalle with tofu, broccoli rabe, dried tomatoes, goat cheese and, **195–97**
    linguine with cilantro, tofu and, **205–6**
    removing kernels from, 197
    tofu and bell pepper fajitas with spicy soybeans, **236–38**
    tofu and white bean burgers, **161–62**
coronary heart disease, see heart disease
couscous, Israeli, 127
    with broccoli rabe and raisins, **278**
    Kate's lentil and chickpea soup with root vegetables and, **125–27**
    poached salmon with vegetables and, **265–66**
    vegetable-beef soup with, **132–34**
cranberry(ies):
    dried, acorn squash stuffed with brown rice, tofu and, **214–15**
    -orange cloud cookies, **293**
    -pecan granola, **119–20**
"creamy" Caesar salad, **173–74**
creamy vanilla-maple sauce, **302–3**
crisps:
    apple and rhubarb, **294–95**
    blueberry, **295–96**

HRT for prevention of, 24, 51, 69–70
risk factors for, 70–71
soy foods for prevention of, 31–32, 69
in women vs. men, 68
herbs and spices, dried, cooking of, 221
high-density lipoprotein (HDL) cholesterol, 24, 41, 42, 51, 68, 69
honey-mustard sauce, tempeh and mozzarella melts with a, **156–57**
hormone replacement therapy (HRT), 47–55
Alzheimer's disease and, 23, 51–52
continuous vs. cyclic methods for, 49
estrogen supplements in, 47–48
making decision on, 54–55
in preventing heart disease, 24, 51, 69–70
progesterone supplements in, 47–48, 49
Raloxifen as alternative to, 53, 65
for relief of menopausal symptoms, 21–22, 49–50
and risk of breast cancer, 52–53, 78–79
and risk of endometrial cancer, 47–48
side effects of, 52
in treating osteoporosis, 23–24, 50–51, 65
hormones:
produced after menopause, 19–20
regulation of, in menopause, 18–19
hot cocoa, **107–8**
hot flashes, 18, 19, 20, 21–22, 25, 26, 53
HRT and, 49–50
soy foods and, 21–22, 29–31
HRT, *see* hormone replacement therapy
hummus:
spicy black bean, **143**
tofu parsley, **142–43**
hydrogenated fat, 39–40

Indian food, 87–88
insomnia, 22, 53

isoflavones, 28–30, 32
Israeli couscous, *see* couscous, Israeli
Italian food, 86–87

jambalaya, **256–57**
Japanese food, 86

kale, collard, and potato soup, **127–28**
Kate's lentil and chickpea soup with root vegetables and couscous, **125–27**

LDL, *see* low-density lipoprotein (LDL) cholesterol
leek(s):
cleaning of, 267
lentil stew with potatoes, goat cheese and, **224–25**
pan-seared tuna with goat cheese, basil and, **266–67**
squash, parsnip, and tofu stew, roasted, **226–27**
lemon:
black bean soup with parsley and, **137–39**
-ginger chicken and tofu, **246–48**
linguine with pepper, tofu, chard and, **200–201**
pan-seared salmon with creamed spinach and, **261–62**
-poppy seed dressing, romaine and mesclun salad with, **170**
pork with capers and, **255–56**
whole-wheat penne with asparagus, chicken and, **197–98**
lentil:
bisque, **129–30**
and chickpea soup with root vegetables and couscous, Kate's, **125–27**
stew with leeks, potatoes, and goat cheese, **224–25**
lignans, 28–29
linguine:
with corn, cilantro, and tofu, **205–6**
with lemon, pepper, tofu, and chard, **200–201**
with littleneck clams, spicy sausage, and tomatoes, **181–82**